Human Pharmacology

HUMAN PHARMACOLOGY

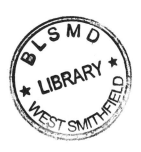
■ Paul Gard

School of Pharmacy and Biomolecular Sciences
University of Brighton, UK

LIFELINES

TAYLOR & FRANCIS
· Founded 1798 ·

London and New York

First published 2001 by Taylor & Francis
11 New Fetter Lane, London EC4P 4EE

Simultaneously published in the USA and Canada
by Taylor & Francis Inc,
29 West 35th Street, New York, NY 10001

Taylor & Francis is an imprint of the Taylor & Francis Group

© 2001 Paul Gard

Typeset in Perpetua and Helvetica by Graphicraft Limited, Hong Kong
Printed and bound in Great Britain by TJ International Ltd, Padstow, Cornwall

British Library Cataloguing in Publication Data
A catalogue record for this book is available from the British Library

Library of Congress Cataloging in Publication Data
Gard, Paul R.
    Human pharmacology / P.R. Gard.
       p.   cm. – (Lifelines in life science)
    Includes bibliographical references and index.
    1. Pharmacology. I. Title. II. Series.
    RM300.G37 2000   00-024000
    615′.1–dc21

ISBN 0–7484–0812–6

CONTENTS

FOREWORD: WHAT IS PHARMACOLOGY AND WHAT DO PHARMACOLOGISTS DO?

Pharmacology is the study of drugs: their development, their use, their adverse effects and their beneficial effects. It is traditionally divided into pharmacodynamics, which studies what the drug does to the body, and pharmacokinetics, which investigates what the body does to the drug. By understanding the nature of the molecular mechanism of drug action, pharmacologists aim to elucidate the underlying cause of disease, to improve upon existing treatments and to discover and develop new treatments for disease. Within the pharmaceutical industry it is the chemists who synthesise potential new drugs but it is then the pharmacologist who tests them for activity. Pharmacologists are responsible for assessing drug efficacy; the possible adverse effects of the drug; the likely effects of overdose; the risks of tolerance and addiction; the speed of onset of action; the duration of action and the route of the drug's metabolism and excretion.

An understanding of pharmacology is also useful for chemists who are engaged in the production of new chemical entities for possible development as medicines; for physiologists, biochemists and psychologists who may use drugs as tools to investigate the normal working of the body; and for anybody involved in the treatment or care of individuals who may be receiving or self-administering drugs, possibly for the prevention or treatment of disease. An understanding of the mechanisms of drug action allows one to predict the effects of the drug, its adverse effects and the possible consequences of overdose. This text aims to provide an introduction to the science of pharmacology and thus to allow the reader to appreciate why and how certain drugs relieve the symptoms of disease.

PRINCIPLES OF DRUG ACTIONS AND EFFECTS

■ 1.1 INTRODUCTION

Pharmacology is the science of drugs. An interesting feature of pharmacology, however, is that although drugs are the focus of attention, the term 'drug' is rarely, if ever, defined. When students of pharmacology are asked for a definition, answers often take the form of 'drugs are chemicals used to treat illness' or 'drugs are chemicals which have an effect on the body'. What these attempted definitions, and others like them, fail to consider is that some drugs are taken by healthy individuals, for example oral contraceptives and recreational drugs, and that many chemicals produce effects on the body, for example dietary constituents, yet dietary proteins and carbohydrates are rarely classified as drugs. One possible definition of a drug would be 'a chemical that alters the normal activity of the body'.

One possible definition of a drug would be 'a chemical that alters the normal activity of the body'

Before the effects of drugs on an individual can be considered, it is first necessary to understand the general principles of how drugs act at a cellular or molecular level to produce changes in the activity of the organism. Equipped with this knowledge, it then becomes easier to appreciate why certain drugs are able to treat certain diseases, why some drugs inevitably cause side-effects and why sometimes the use of two drugs in combination can inadvertently reduce the ability of those drugs to treat a disease because of mutual interference.

■ 1.2 THE DOSE–RESPONSE RELATIONSHIP

Most people recognise that the effect of a given drug can be increased by raising the dose that is administered. Thus if alcohol (ethanol) is used as an example, at low doses there is no significant effect but as the dose increases the degree of intoxication increases; intoxication induced by ethanol is thus said to be a graded response. This increase in intoxication, however, is not linear, thus drinking an eighth glass of beer does not cause the same (absolute) increase in drunkenness as did drinking the third glass. The hyperbolic nature of the dose–response relationship is presented in figure 1.1. Another feature of alcohol intoxication is the limit of its response: at high doses ethanol can be lethal. At these doses, an increase in dose will not induce an increase in response, it is impossible to become 'more dead'. Thus, as portrayed in figure 1.1, there is a maximal response to ethanol. All drugs have limits to the response that they can elicit, although usually this maximal response is not death!

At high doses ethanol can be lethal, at this point an increase in dose will not induce an increase in response; it is impossible to become 'more dead'

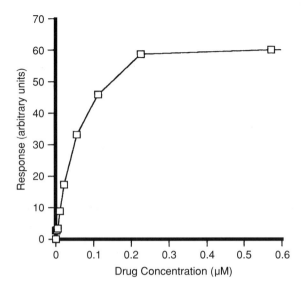

• **Figure 1.1** A representation of the typical relationship between concentration (dose) of drug used and the size of the response elicited

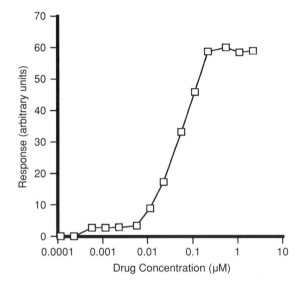

• **Figure 1.2** A logarithmic transformation of the concentration–response curve shown in figure 1.1, showing how the log dose–response curve allows a wider range of concentrations to be plotted, and results in a sigmoid curve, the central portion of which is approximately linear

A logarithmic transformation of the dose–response curve produces a curve, the central portion of which approximates to a straight line

With the advent of computers it has been easier to determine the mathematical equation of the dose–response curve; however, in the early days of pharmacology such computations were more troublesome. The original descriptions of the drug concentration–response relationship noted that a logarithmic transformation of the data produced a sigmoid ('S-shaped') curve, the central portion of which approximated to a straight line (figure 1.2). It is because of the relative ease of handling data with a straight line relationship that it became conventional to portray the relationship using log concentration or log dose–response curves; these logarithmic curves also allow a wide range of doses to be plotted on the same axes.

In many cases drugs produce more than one response; thus, for example, ethanol not only produces effects on the central nervous system (CNS) which results in decreased co-ordination, but there may also be flushing (reddening of the face and neck). The dose–response relationship for flushing is different to that for CNS depression. In the

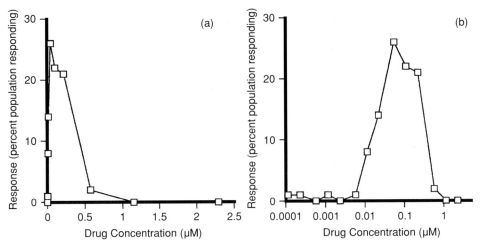

• **Figure 1.3** A representation of the typical relationship between (a) the dose (concentration) of drug used and the proportion of the population that exhibits a quantal response. (b) A logarithmic transformation of graph (a) results in a distribution curve which approximates to the normal distribution

therapeutic arena this means that it may be possible to increase the dose of drug being used in order to increase the desired response, but that there will not necessarily be an increase in some other effect because the maximal response for the secondary response may have already been achieved. The ability of a drug to produce an effect, and the dose required, is sometimes expressed as the EC_{50}, Effective Concentration: 50%. This value represents the concentration of drug required to produce a response which is 50% of the maximal response. Related values are the ED_{50} (Effective Dose: 50%) and IC_{50} (Inhibitory Concentration: 50%), the concentration required to reduce a variable (for example heart rate) to 50% of its normal value.

Quantal responses are 'all or nothing', for example a patient is either 'dead' or 'alive'

Some drug responses are classified as quantal rather than graded. Quantal responses are 'all or nothing' responses, an example of such a response is death: an individual is either dead or alive, one cannot be half dead. Other examples of quantal responses include the effects of drugs on nerve impulses: a local anaesthetic drug either prevents a nerve action potential or it doesn't; in general anaesthesia the level of anaesthesia may be assessed using the corneal response (blink reflex) – stimulation of the cornea either elicits a blink response or it doesn't. The classification of graded or quantal is a property of the response rather than of the drug; however, graded responses may sometimes be converted to quantal responses by application of a 'cut-off' criterion. An example of such a conversion would be in the assessment of the effects of ethanol on balance. An experimenter may attempt to grade or rate balance on a scale of 1 to 10 using a variety of measurements or, alternatively, he may simply record the dose of ethanol required to cause loss of balance (i.e. 'falling over'). The response has thus been converted from a graded response to a quantal response. Within a given population, different individuals will require different doses to elicit the response, figure 1.3a indicates the relationship between the dose and the proportion of the population responding. A logarithmic transformation of the dose produces a curve which approximates to a normal distribution (figure 1.3b). The final feature, depicted in figure 1.4, is biological variation. People may respond differently to a given dose of drug for a variety of reasons (see Chapter 10). Reasons for biological variation in responses to drugs include tolerance, where repeated use of a drug by an individual induces a gradual reduction in the size of the response seen, and tachyphylaxis, where the effect of the drug decreases markedly after only the first or second dose (see later).

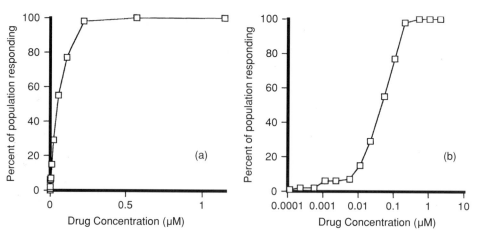

• **Figure 1.4** A typical graph showing how the relationship between the dose (concentration) of drug used and the proportion of the population exhibiting a quantal response, when plotted cumulatively, resembles (a) the concentration–response curve for a graded response, and (b) the log concentration–response curve for a graded response

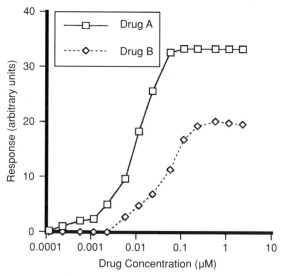

• **Figure 1.5** A representation of the log concentration–response curves for different drugs, showing how different drugs may produce different maximal effects, and may require different concentrations (doses) to produce those effects

At first glance the use of a quantal response appears to render dose–response curves unusable as at low doses there is no effect, at a given dose the effect occurs but at higher doses the magnitude of the effect remains unchanged. But if the ability of a drug to elicit a quantal response is studied in a population, the results, when expressed in a cumulative manner, resemble the classic log dose–response curve described above (figure 1.4). Such a representation again allows the drug actions to be expressed in terms of the ED_{50}, but in this case the dose referred to is that dose which is effective in 50% of the population (see above for definition of ED_{50} for a graded response). Related values for quantal responses are LD_{50} (Lethal Dose: 50%), the dose required to kill 50% of the test population, and LD_{10} (Lethal Dose: 10%), the dose required to kill 10% of the test population.

The LD_{50} is the dose required to kill 50% of the test population

It is by using dose or log dose–response curves that the properties of different drugs can be compared. Figure 1.5 illustrates that some drugs are able to produce responses at lower doses than others; such drugs are said to be more potent. It is often assumed that drugs of higher potency are of greater therapeutic value but, all other things being equal (i.e. adverse effects, etc.), this belief is erroneous. Unless the dose of drug that is prescribed is uncomfortably large to take, it makes no difference to the recipient whether he or she is required to take 1mg of one drug or 100mg of another. It should be remembered that tablets invariably contain a large proportion of excipients. Excipients are those pharmacologically inert substances added to tablets to act as bulking agents, to facilitate the manufacturing process and to affect drug absorption, etc. A tablet containing 300mg of aspirin may thus weigh 1.3g, it would therefore be possible to increase the amount of drug contained within a tablet without having much effect on its final weight. Another drug property that influences its therapeutic usefulness is its maximal response; as shown in figure 1.5, some drugs elicit greater responses than others. An example of this would be the ability of aspirin and morphine to relieve pain. Both aspirin and morphine could be used to relieve the pain of toothache; however, no matter what dose was offered, few people would be willing to undergo abdominal surgery with aspirin as the only form of pain relief. Surgery could be performed with the aid of morphine. This example illustrates how the maximal response to a drug may limit its uses, but also shows that a low maximal response, in itself, does not negate a drug's usefulness.

A drug's maximal effect may limit its uses, but a low maximal effect does not negate its usefulness

■ 1.3 MECHANISMS OF DRUG ACTION

In some cases the effects of a drug are dependent solely upon its physicochemical properties. The archetypal example of such a drug would be an antacid used for the relief of indigestion or to promote healing of a gastric ulcer. In terms of pharmacology, the only important feature of such drugs is their pH, they must be alkaline in order to neutralise the acid pH of the stomach. Any form of alkali would work, although, of course, other considerations such as toxic effects and the quantities required must be taken into account.

Osmotic diuretics are another class of drug where the actions are dependent upon the general physicochemical properties. Diuretics are drugs that are used to increase the volume of urine excreted; osmotic diuretics act because they are not metabolised at all by the body and are thus excreted, unchanged, via the urine. Because of their osmotic properties, as these diuretics are excreted they take water with them by osmosis, thus causing a net loss of fluid (see Chapter 4).

A slight change in chemical structure may render a drug inactive

For most drugs their action is dependent upon their precise chemical structure. A slight change in chemical structure, for example the addition of an extra methyl sidechain or the removal of a ketone group, may render the drug inactive. This specificity of drug action can be explained by use of the concept of receptors. In the early years of this century it was proposed that the body possesses certain receptors or receptor substances and that drugs combine with these receptors to produce their effects. Individual drugs are only able to interact with certain receptors, and individual subtypes of receptors can only be stimulated by certain drugs. Pharmacology then borrowed from enzyme biochemistry to develop the 'lock and key' hypothesis of drug action. A cell's receptor can be envisaged as a lock, thus the drug is the key that can open the lock. The drug must be of the correct shape (chemical structure) for it to be able to fit into the receptor. In this way it becomes apparent why a relatively minor change in the chemical structure of a drug may render it unable to interact with its receptor (figure 1.6). This hypothesis would

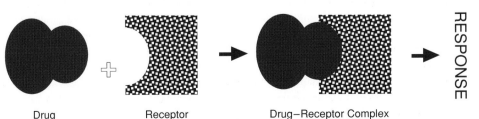

Drug   Receptor   Drug–Receptor Complex   RESPONSE

• **Figure 1.6** A schematic representation of the 'lock and key hypothesis' of drug–receptor interactions, illustrating the mechanism of action of agonist drugs

• **Figure 1.7** A representation of drug–receptor interactions in the form of a quasi chemical equation

$$[\text{DRUG}] + [\text{RECEPTOR}] \underset{k_{-1}}{\overset{k_1}{\rightleftharpoons}} [\text{DRUG–RECEPTOR COMPLEX}] \xrightarrow{\text{Intrinsic activity}} \text{RESPONSE}$$

k_1 = Association Constant
k_{-1} = Dissociation Constant

$\dfrac{k_1}{k_{-1}}$ = Affinity (K_A)

There are 15–20,000 drugs available for therapeutic use, but only 150 therapeutically important human 'drug' receptors

suggest that every single drug requires its own receptor, and that each cell must have receptors to that drug if it is to respond. This is not true, there are 15–20,000 drugs currently available for therapeutic use; however, there are only approximately 150 therapeutically important types of human drug receptor, this indicates that many different drugs must be able to share the same receptor.

Receptors are proteins that are synthesised by the cell in the same way as any other proteins are synthesised. The synthesis of these receptor proteins is under genetic control, thus all cells have the ability to synthesise all receptors; however, variations in the extent of gene expression means that an individual cell (or tissue) may only synthesise receptors for three or four different messengers. It can therefore be seen why drugs are only able to produce effects on selected target tissues. It has been shown that cells that do express a particular type of receptor may each possess in the region of several thousand of those receptors. The nature of receptors is described later.

Use of the concept of receptors, and the lock and key hypothesis allows the dose–response relationship to be viewed in more quantitative terms. It is known that the response to a drug is proportional to the amount (dose or concentration) of drug present. This can now be modified such that the size of the response is proportional to the number of drug–receptor interactions (figure 1.7). It can therefore be seen that the size of response will be limited by the number of receptors available. The other variable that will influence the size of response for a given drug concentration is the 'ease' with which the drug and receptor interacts. If figure 1.7 is considered as a chemical equation, k_1 is the association rate constant, i.e. the ease with which the drug and the receptor bind together, and k_{-1} is the dissociation rate constant, the ease with which the drug and receptor later separate. The net result of the k_1 and the k_{-1} determines how much drug is bound to its receptors at any one time. This parameter is usually called the affinity, and it can be viewed as the 'goodness of fit' of a drug for its receptor.

Experimental data, however, fail to fit the simple hypothesis that the size of the response to a given drug is dependent upon the affinity of the drug for its receptor and the number of receptors occupied, the maximal response being obtained when all of the receptors are occupied. First, it was noted that a maximal response can sometimes be achieved with less than 100% receptor occupation. This gave rise to the concept of spare receptors, i.e. that the system possesses more receptors than are actually required. The molecular basis of this is discussed later in this chapter. The second departure from the simple view came from the observation that two drugs, at equal concentrations, with identical affinities for their mutual receptor, produced different sizes of response. This gave rise to the concept of 'intrinsic activity' or 'efficacy' (two terms used interchangeably).

There are no units for intrinsic activity; its either high or low

There are no units for intrinsic activity, it is simply a concept to explain why some drugs produce smaller responses than would otherwise be expected: 'low intrinsic activity'.

There is a particular group of drugs which have affinity for their receptor but have an intrinsic activity of zero, hence they are unable to produce a response at any concentra-

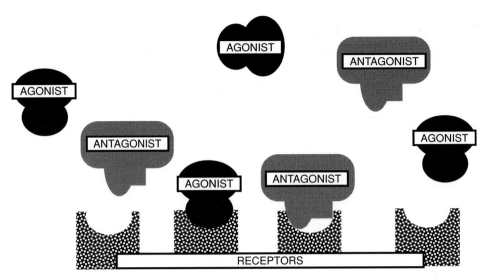

• **Figure 1.8** A schematic representation of the 'lock and key hypothesis' illustrating the competition of agonists and antagonists for the receptor

tion. The important feature of these drugs is that they bind to the receptor, and in so doing prevent access to that receptor for other drugs which do have intrinsic activity. Such drugs are called antagonists, they elicit no response other than preventing the actions of other drugs. Drugs which possess intrinsic activity are called agonists. Thus antagonists are able to prevent, or reduce, the responses to agonists. Drugs with very low intrinsic activity are partial agonists: they bind to the receptor and produce a small response, but in so doing they deny access of full agonists to the receptor. Partial agonists can be viewed as antagonists with slight agonist properties.

Antagonists do not produce a response other than to prevent the actions of other drugs or messengers

The effects of an antagonist on the responses induced by an agonist are dependent upon the nature of the interaction of the antagonist with the receptor, and the relative affinities of the agonist and antagonist. Figure 1.8 illustrates that if the agonist and antagonist bind to the receptor at the same points and with approximately equal affinities then competitive antagonism ensues. This means that the number of receptors occupied by agonist and the number occupied by antagonist are primarily dependent on the relative concentrations of the two chemicals. Thus at lower relative concentrations of antagonist, most receptors will be occupied by agonist, but at higher relative concentrations of antagonist most receptors will be occupied by antagonist, hence the size of the response will be greatly reduced. Even in the presence of a high concentration of antagonist, however, the proportion of receptors occupied by agonist can be increased by increasing the relative concentration of agonist. Thus it is always possible to obtain a maximal response to an agonist, even in the presence of a competitive antagonist, simply by increasing the concentration of agonist. Competitive antagonism is therefore sometimes also known as surmountable antagonism. Because the presence of antagonist means that a higher concentration of agonist is required to produce the same size response, the antagonist is said to have decreased the apparent affinity of the agonist for its receptor, graphically this effect produces a parallel shift of the log dose–response curve to the right (figure 1.9). The relative potencies of competitive antagonists can be expressed in terms of pA_2 values, see Box 1.1.

It is always possible to elicit a maximal response in the presence of a competitive antagonist by increasing the dose of agonist

If the antagonist interacts with the receptor at a site different from that acted upon by the agonist, sometimes called an allosteric binding site, the process is termed non-competitive antagonism. With this form of antagonism, once the antagonist interacts with

• **Figure 1.9** A graphical representation of the effects of different concentrations of a competitive antagonist on the responses induced by an agonist

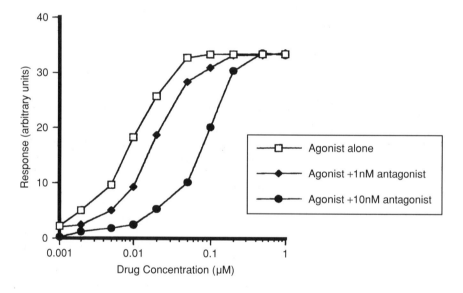

Non-competitive antagonism is insurmountable

the receptor it can not be displaced, or otherwise overcome, by the agonist. Non-competitive antagonists thus effectively remove the receptor from the system; however, those receptors which remain unaffected by the antagonist are still available for inter-action with the agonist. This form of antagonism has the effect of decreasing the maximal response that can be produced by the agonist and causing a 'collapse' of the log dose–response curve (figure 1.10). More advanced theories to explain the effects of agonists and antagonists are presented in Box 1.2.

■ 1.4 THE NATURE OF RECEPTORS

It may initially seem odd that the body possesses receptors for what are, in many cases, man-made drugs. Why should the body have the inherent ability to respond to heroin: a chemical related to opium, an extract of a poppy? In most cases, however, the drugs are mimicking or modifying (i.e. antagonising) the effects of one of the body's natural trans-mitter substances, such as a neurotransmitter or a hormone. Thus the body possesses receptors as part of its own control processes; at times of illness the symptoms that arise usually reflect an abnormality in one of those control processes, hence the job of the

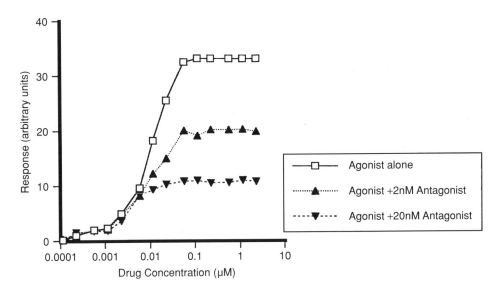

• **Figure 1.10** A graphical representation of the effects of different concentrations of a non-competitive antagonist on the responses induced by an agonist

---

■ *Box 1.2* Theories of drug receptor action

The 'lock and key' hypothesis is the simplest hypothesis to explain drug action; however, this hypothesis is not able to explain all experimental observations. Early modifications of the hypothesis led to the development of contradictory theories: occupation theory and rate theory. Occupation theory stated that the response obtained was proportional to the number of receptors occupied, whereas rate theory stated that the response was dependent on the rate of drug–receptor interactions. For the occupation theory, drugs which dissociated from the receptor only slowly (i.e. low dissociation rate constant) would be expected to produce greater responses than drugs which rapidly vacated the receptor. Conversely, the rate theory would expect drugs with high dissociation rate constants to leave the receptor rapidly, thus making it available for further stimulation by other molecules of agonist. Experimental results generally show that high K_{-1} is associated with high potency, thus supporting rate theory.

A further model for drug–receptor interactions is the two-state theory. This theory states that a receptor can exist in two separate states: active and inactive. These two states are in dynamic equilibrium; however, the inactive state may predominate in the absence of agonist. If a drug has a higher affinity for the active state it will preferentially bind to that state, and in doing so shift the equilibrium away from the inactive state, such a drug would act as an agonist. Drugs which bind equally to both receptor states would stabilize the receptor in its inactive state, but would not prevent the ability of an agonist to shift the equilibrium. Such drugs would be competitive antagonists. Some drugs may bind preferentially to the inactive state of the receptor, thus shifting the equilibrium towards the inactive state. Such drugs produce effects opposite to the effects produced by agonists and are called inverse agonists.

---

pharmacologist is to identify which receptors are involved in the production of the symptoms, and to develop drugs for the relief of those symptoms. Ironically, there are some receptors that have been identified for which the endogenous ligand is unknown, and for which the physiological function is unclear, these receptors are called orphan receptors.

In most cases drugs mimic or modify the actions of the body's endogenous transmitters

The body possesses many different hormones, local hormones (autocoids) and neurotransmitters, each of which has its own receptors; in many cases there are different subtypes of receptor for individual messengers. It follows, therefore, that there are several hundred different types of receptor. Fortunately, it is possible to divide the receptors into different subtypes. The first form of receptor classification is based upon the site of the receptor within the cell. Some receptors are located within the cell cytoplasm or within the nucleus. In order for the drug to interact with these receptors it must first cross the lipid cell membrane. Lipid-soluble drugs, such as the anabolic steroids (see Chapter 8), are able to cross the cell membrane readily, thus they are able to interact with intracellular receptors. In the absence of specific membrane transport mechanisms, however, water-soluble drugs are unable to cross the cell membrane, thus they are unable to interact with intracellular receptors. In the case of these drugs they can only interact with receptors that are held within the cell membrane, with that part of the receptor that interacts with the drug being outside of the cell; the drugs are thus able to interact with the receptor without the necessity of ever crossing the cell membrane or entering the cell. These receptors traverse the cell membrane and therefore have some parts in direct contact with the cytoplasm. It is because these receptors span the cell membrane that the interaction of a drug with a receptor outside the cell is able to produce an effect inside the cell.

■ 1.4.1 INTRACELLULAR RECEPTORS

1.4.1.1 Deoxyribonucleic acid (DNA)

Deoxyribonucleic acid (DNA) carries all of the genetic material of the cell and at times of cell division it replicates itself and is thus passed on to all offspring cells. DNA, via ribonucleic acid (RNA), is responsible for protein synthesis. Certain anticancer agents, for example the alkylating agents and cisplatin, are able to enter the cell and the nucleus and bind to specific regions (base nucleic acids) of DNA, often strongly linking the two DNA strands together. In doing so these drugs prevent the DNA strands from 'unzipping' and replicating, and hence prevent the growth of rapidly dividing tissues such as tumours (figure 1.11). The major problem with this type of drug is that they are non-selective in their action, thus they also prevent the division of other cells, such as hair

• **Figure 1.11** A schematic representation of the interaction between an anticancer drug and the double helix of deoxyribonucleic acid (DNA)

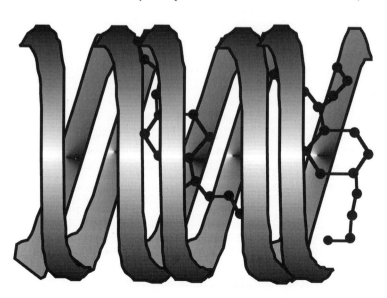

and spermatocytes, thus producing the well-known adverse effects of these anticancer therapies.

1.4.1.2 Intracellular enzymes

In a way similar to that described above, some drugs interact with specific regions of the protein matrix of enzymes. By doing this the drug may occupy the active site of the enzyme, thus preventing the enzyme's ability to perform its role as a biochemical catalyst; in some cases the drug acts as a false substrate for the enzyme, resulting in the synthesis of an inactive product. If the usual substrate for that enzyme is able to displace the drug, such enzyme inhibition would be competitive, and reversible. In some cases the drug binds to regions of the enzyme protein which are distant from the normal active site; however, such an interaction may produce conformational changes in the protein which render the enzyme inactive (allosteric effect). Such an effect would render the drug a non-competitive enzyme inhibitor.

1.4.1.3 Steroid hormone receptors

A major group of intracellular receptors are those that normally interact with the steroid hormones such as testosterone and the androgens (Chapter 8), although similar receptors interact with non-steroid messengers such as thyroid hormones. The normal function of these receptors is to influence gene expression and protein synthesis. The receptor protein enters the nucleus and binds to a region of the DNA called the hormone response element, the effect of which is to influence processes such as gene expression and RNA transcription (figure 1.12). The receptor alone is only weakly able to perform this role, but in the presence of the hormone the hormone–receptor complex is much more effective, hence hormones may profoundly alter (increase or decrease) the rate of synthesis of a particular protein, or may initiate the synthesis of a novel protein. In some cases the receptor normally resides within the cytoplasm and only migrates to the nucleus when bound to the appropriate hormone, in other cases the receptor normally resides within the nucleus. For interaction with these receptors drugs must be able to cross the cell membrane, usually by simple diffusion of the lipid-soluble drug through the membrane, but in some cases there is evidence of a carrier-mediated transport process. The drugs may be either agonists of the hormone receptor, in which case they mimic the effects of

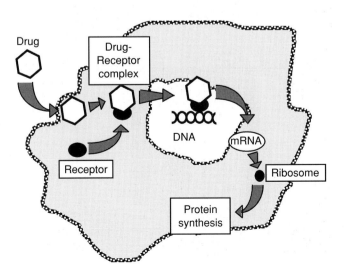

• Figure 1.12 An illustration of the mechanism of action of steroid hormones and drugs, acting via intracellular receptors

Drugs acting on intracellular receptors usually have long-lasting effects which are slow to onset

the hormone, or they may be antagonists of the receptor, in which case they reduce or prevent hormonal action. Because drugs acting on these receptors cause an increase or decrease in the rate of synthesis of a particular protein, or may initiate the synthesis of a novel protein, the drugs' effects tend to be slow in onset, but long lasting.

■ 1.4.2 MEMBRANE BOUND RECEPTORS

Within the group of receptors classified as membrane-bound receptors there are different subgroups of receptors, each of which utilises a different mechanism to produce a change in the intracellular environment and ultimately cellular activity. The four broad subgroups of membrane-bound drug receptors are: ion channels, carrier proteins, membrane-bound enzymes and G-protein coupled receptors.

1.4.2.1 Ion channels

Anchored within the lipid layers of the cell membrane are pores or channels that allow the exchange of ions or water between the cytoplasm and the extracellular fluid, these ion channels are vital in the control of cell volume and the activity of electrically excitable cells. Ion channels are composed of proteins that span the cell membrane and are arranged in such a manner that they form a hollow protein cylinder through which ions may pass (figure 1.13). Typically the pores are not constantly open, but rather they open or close in response to various stimuli. Probably the best-known example of the opening and closing of ion channels occurs during the propagation of an action potential along a nerve fibre. Under resting conditions the sodium–potassium pump (Na^+,K^+-ATPase) expels sodium from the interior of the cell, thus causing the inside of the cell to be electrically

• **Figure 1.13** A diagrammatic representation of an ion channel; conformation changes within the protein cylinders of the channel lead to opening or closing of the pore. Some drugs bind to sites on the extracellular surface of the ion channel to influence channel opening and closing, other drugs influence channel opening following interaction with a G-protein coupled receptor

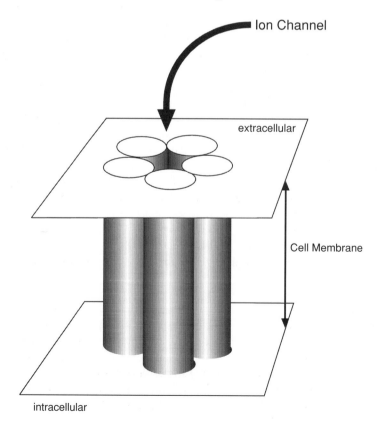

Ion Channel

extracellular

Cell Membrane

intracellular

negative with respect to the outside. A change in the transmembrane potential from the normal resting value of −60mV (with respect to the inside of the cell) to a value of about −20mV results in the brief opening of sodium ion channels. The result of this is an influx of sodium from the high concentrations outside of the cell to the lower concentrations inside the cell. This increase in the number of positively charged sodium ions entering the cell means that the membrane potential changes further and may reach a value of approximately +20mV before the sodium ion channels close. This further change in membrane potential, however, also causes the opening of separate potassium ion channels, which results in the movement of potassium ions from the high intracellular concentrations to the lower extracellular concentrations. The efflux of positively charged potassium ions from the inside of the cell means that the membrane potential becomes more negative and eventually regains its resting potential of −60mV. Such ionic movements, and their consequences, form the basis of nerve actions and muscle contraction. In the current context, the important feature of this process is the demonstration that the opening and closing of the ion channels is dependent upon the transmembrane electrical potential. Such ion channels are termed voltage-gated ion channels; however, there are certain drugs which are able to interfere with the activity of these voltage-gated ion channels: local anaesthetic drugs (Chapter 2), for example, bind to the protein of the ion channel and in doing so block the ionic pore. In this case the protein of the voltage-gated ion channel is itself acting as the drug receptor.

A ligand is a chemical that binds selectively to another chemical, such as a receptor

Members of the second group of ion channels are called ligand-gated ion channels. A ligand is a chemical that will interact or bind selectively to another chemical, in this case a chemical that will bind selectively to an ion channel or receptor. Again, these ligand-gated ion channels are hollow protein cylinders which span the cell membrane and allow the passage of ions. Unlike voltage-gated channels, the stimulus for the opening of a ligand-gated channel is the presence of the appropriate ligand and the interaction of that ligand with the protein of the ion channel. The nicotinic acetylcholine receptor of the neuromuscular junction is an example of a ligand-gated ion channel. In the presence of the messenger acetylcholine, the ion channel opens, thus permitting the passage of sodium and potassium ions, ultimately inducing a muscle contraction.

A third example of a drug receptor being directly associated with an ion channel is a subtype of the receptor for γ-aminobutyric acid (GABA), the predominant inhibitory neurotransmitter in the human brain. The GABA type A receptor is linked to a chloride ion channel, thus the action of GABA is to open the channel, allowing chloride ions to enter the cell, which makes it more difficult for the cell to depolarise. Drugs such as barbiturates and benzodiazepines (Chapter 3) bind to the ion channel protein at a site distant from the GABA recognition (binding) site, but they influence the effects of GABA, potentiating its effects. Such distant recognition sites are referred to as allosteric receptors. The resultant effect of barbiturates and benzodiazepines is to make the cells even less excitable, thus they can be used as sedatives or in the treatment of convulsions (e.g. epilepsy).

Binding sites distinct from the agonist binding site are called allosteric receptors

1.4.2.2 Carrier proteins
Lipid-soluble chemicals are able to cross the cell membrane by simple diffusion; however, this is not possible for hydrophilic moieties. Many cells, however, possess carriers that are able to transport chemicals across the cell membrane, often against the concentration gradient. Examples of such carriers include those for glucose and amino acid uptake into cells, as well as the carrier mechanisms involved in kidney function (Chapter 5) and the inactivation of certain neurotransmitters (Chapter 3). These carrier mechanisms

are often susceptible to the actions of drugs, thereby resulting in an alteration of the normal cellular activity.

1.4.2.3 Membrane-bound enzymes

Another group of membrane-bound receptors are the kinase receptors, such as tyrosine kinase receptors and serine–threonine kinase receptors. An important feature of these receptors is that the receptor protein itself is an enzyme, thus interaction of the extracellular portion of the receptor with the messenger or drug causes a change in the enzymic activity of the intracellular portion. The ultimate effect of the activation of these receptors is usually a stimulation of anabolic processes such as protein synthesis, growth and metabolism, drugs acting via these receptors are therefore generally slower in action than drugs acting on ion channel receptors, but they are faster than drugs acting via intracellular receptors.

The largest group of receptors of this type are the tyrosine kinase receptors, these receptors generally have a single protein chain which spans the cell membrane, although in several cases the chains dimerize to form a symetrical receptor which requires two molecules of agonist for activation. The endogenous ligands for tyrosine kinase receptors are usually hormones and upon stimulation of the receptor by the hormone the receptors phosphorylate certain regulatory proteins (for example phospholipase C), specifically on the tyrosine hydroxyl terminals; importantly the receptor is able to induce phosphorylation of tyrosine residues of its own protein structure. One result of the protein phosphorylation is an alteration of the activity of the regulatory protein; thus, for example, autophosphorylation of the receptor protein leads to an increase in receptor activity. Another result of the phosphorylation of regulatory proteins is that they then interact with growth factor receptors to provide a focus for the binding, and subsequents actions, of various growth factors. In many cases this chain of events results in the activation of a membrane-bound enzyme called ras (which is normally bound to guanosine diphosphate in a manner similar to G-proteins, see Section 1.4.2.5), and ultimately the activation of mitogen-activated protein kinase (MAPK). MAPK is a serine–threonine protein kinase (see later) which migrates from the cytoplasm to the nucleus where it interacts with a number of proteins to influence gene expression and cell proliferation.

A similar group of receptors are the serine–threonine kinase receptors, which again are normally activated by hormones. These receptors also regulate growth and differentiation. Serine–threonine kinase receptors are normally composed of two protein chains which span the cell membrane once. The intracellular portion of each chain possesses serine–threonine kinase activity, but the two chains usually perform separate functions. The first chain acts as the extracellular hormone binding site, and its stimulation results in phosphorylation of the serine–threonine residues of the second protein chain. The activation of the second protein chain results in the alteration of the activity of various nuclear regulatory proteins, culminating in regulation of mitogenesis and differentiation. Serine–threonine receptors are longer acting than tyrosine kinase receptors.

Tyrosine kinase receptors and serine–threonine kinase receptors influence cell differentiation and division

1.4.2.4 Guanyl cyclase receptors

These receptors are single protein chains which possess both enzymic activity and a ligand-binding domain. The receptors may be either intracellular or membrane bound. Activation of the protein catalyses the formation of cyclic guanosine monophosphate (cGMP) from guanosine triphosphate (GTP), the cGMP then activates a series of serine–threonine protein kinases which phosphorylate other intracellular proteins, thus regulating their activity.

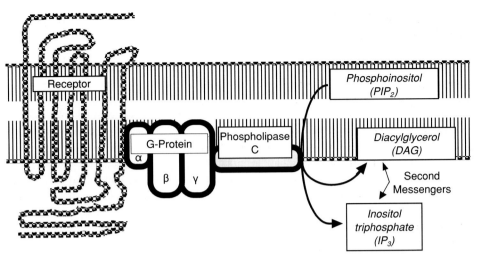

• **Figure 1.14** An illustration of the protein structure of a 'seven transmembrane domain' receptor and its interaction, via the G-protein, with enzymes responsible for the synthesis of second messengers

1.4.2.5 G-protein coupled receptors

The common feature of this group of drug receptors is that they all utilise a protein called G-protein, so called because of its interaction with guanosine triphosphate (GTP) and guanosine diphosphate (GDP). The other common feature is their similar structure. These receptors are all long-chain proteins comprised of 350–600 amino acids which are folded in a 'concertina-like' fashion such that they cross the cell membrane seven times (figure 1.14). These receptors are said to have 'seven transmembrane domains'. The amino end of the protein remains extracellular whereas the carboxylic end, which is intracellular, interacts with the G-protein, which is bound to the intracellular surface of the cell membrane. When the appropriate drug interacts with the ligand-binding domain of the receptor protein, which is on the extracellular aspect of one of the transmembrane helices, a conformation change in the receptor protein takes place such that the intracellular end stimulates the G-protein. In this way the drug is able to induce a change inside the target cell without itself having to enter the cell.

The G-protein is made up of three subunits, the α-subunit, which is linked to the receptor protein, and the β- and γ-subunits. To date nearly 20 different α-subunits have been identified, with six different β- and 11 different γ-subunits, there are therefore many different combinations possible. The G-protein α-subunits exist in two states: an inactive state, in which it is bound to guanosine diphosphate (GDP), and an active state, in which it is bound to guanosine triphosphate (GTP). The α-subunit itself, however, possesses intrinsic GTPase activity and so converts GTP to GDP, thus it normally returns itself to the inactive state. When the receptor is stimulated, the α-subunit dissociates both from its βγ-subunit and from the bound GDP; the GDP is then replaced by GTP. The fate of the separated βγ-subunit will be described later, but while the α-subunit is coupled to GTP, i.e. in its activated state, it is able to interact with one of several adjacent membrane-bound proteins. Examples of such proteins are the enzymes adenylyl cyclase and phospholipase C (PLC) and certain potassium and calcium ion channels. The uncoupled βγ-subunit also has the ability to interact with adenylyl cyclase and PLC and ion channels, although often the α- and βγ-subunits interact with different proteins. The effect of the receptor stimulation ceases when the α-subunit catalyses the conversion of the bound GTP to GDP, thus returning itself to the inactive state, when it re-associates with the βγ-subunit. It should be remembered, however, that because it takes time

G-protein coupled receptors all have seven transmembrane domains

Activation of the G-protein means that an ion channel may be open for several seconds

for the α-subunit to convert GTP to GDP (up to several seconds) the influence of the receptor stimulation on the membrane-bound enzyme or the ion channel is relatively long lasting.

The α-subunits can be divided into four families: the G_s family, which stimulates adenylyl cyclase; the G_i family, which inhibits adenylyl cyclase, this family also contains G_0 which is linked to ion channels; the G_q family, which stimulates PLC; and the $G_{12/13}$ family, which is linked to ion channels. No G-protein α-subunit is known to inhibit PLC.

The consequence of the stimulation of adenylyl cyclase is the conversion of adenosine triphosphate (ATP) to cyclic adenosine monophosphate (cyclic AMP or cAMP). The released cAMP is then able to act within the cell in which it is produced, but because of its hydrophilic nature it is unable to cross the lipid cell membrane and leave that cell. Cyclic AMP is an example of a second messenger. The first messenger is the endogenous ligand for the receptor or the drug; however, because these are unable to cross the cell membrane they require the use of a second messenger to influence processes within the cell. Once produced, the cAMP activates enzymes called cAMP-dependent protein kinases. These second enzymes alter the activity of key intracellular regulatory proteins, such as enzymes, by their phosphorylation of serine–threonine residues; cAMP-dependent protein kinases may also phosphorylate serine–threonine residues of certain ion channels. Depending upon the regulatory protein concerned, the phosphorylation may result in either activation or inhibition. In this way, the stimulation of a G-protein coupled receptor may result in either an increase or a decrease in the activity of the target cell or tissue. The action of cAMP is terminated by its metabolism by the intracellular enzyme phosphodiesterase, of which there are several subtypes.

The consequence of the stimulation of PLC by the G-protein coupled receptor is the catalysis of the hydrolysis of phosphoinositides, which are phospholipids normally found within the cell membrane. This results in the production of inositol triphosphate (IP_3) and diacylglycerol (DAG), both of which act as second messengers. Like cAMP, these two second messengers influence the activity of intracellular enzymes by causing their phosphorylation. IP_3 acts by binding to a specific IP_3 receptor in the endoplasmic reticulum, to release calcium ions. This in turn activates calcium- and calmodulin-dependent protein kinases with results similar to those described for cAMP. Unlike cAMP and IP_3, DAG is lipid soluble, thus it remains within the cell membrane where it stimulates a subtype of protein kinase, called protein kinase C, which, like the other protein kinases, catalyses the phosphorylation of regulatory proteins such as enzymes. Some texts suggest that the lipid solubility of DAG enables it to leave the cell in which it was produced, possibly to influence adjacent cells. It can therefore be seen how the interaction of a ligand with a G-protein coupled receptor results in a change in cellular activity.

Several other features of G-protein coupled receptors remain to be described. First, it is not unusual for several different types of receptor, in a single cell, all to be associated with a single G-protein, association of two receptors of the same type with a single G-protein would explain the phenomenon of spare receptors (see Section 1.3). Conversely, a single receptor may interact with more than one G-protein, and hence utilise two different second messengers. This, together with the fact that the same second messenger may be regulated by several different G-proteins means that there is an 'in-built' intracellular co-ordination of the incoming stimuli. Another feature of the system is its role as an amplifier. Because the G-protein may remain stimulated for several seconds, it is able to catalyse many reactions, thus a single ligand (or drug)–receptor interaction may result in the generation of over 1000 molecules of second messenger.

Activation of the G-proteins results in alterations in the synthesis of the second messengers cAMP and IP3

A single agonist–receptor interaction may result in the synthesis of over 1000 molecules of second messenger

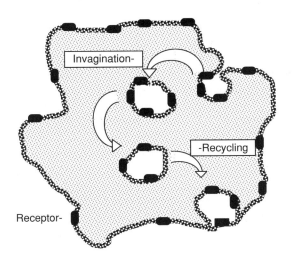

• **Figure 1.15** A diagrammatic representation of receptor down-regulation following invagination of membrane fragments

■ 1.5 VARIATIONS IN RECEPTOR DISTRIBUTION AND POPULATION

As already described, some intracellular receptors may repeatedly move between the cytoplasm and the nucleus, dependent upon their state of activation. Similarly, activation of a steroid receptor may either increase or, more commonly, decrease the expression of that or another receptor. Thus it can be seen that a given receptor population is not constant, and that the activity of a drug may be influenced not only by the concentrations of circulating drug, but also by the state of the receptor population.

In the case of the membrane-bound receptors, it has been shown that these receptors are able to migrate across the cell surface but that they are held within the plane of the cell membrane, and may congregate in clusters of receptors of a similar type. It has also been observed that sections of cell membrane containing drug receptors may invaginate to produce vesicles. This may occur following binding of the drug to the receptor, where it is a mechanism by which the drug is rapidly dissociated from the receptor. The drug may then be broken down by intracellular enzymes while the receptor is recirculated to the membrane, ready for restimulation. However, this may also occur to unbound receptors. It has been postulated that at times of excessive receptor stimulation the cell membrane invaginates, taking with it receptors, and therefore reduces the extent of the response to the circulating drug or transmitter concentration (figure 1.15). Invagination may occur following repeated stimulation of that receptor by an agonist, or it may occur following stimulation of another receptor. While in the vesicles, the receptors may be susceptible to breakdown by enzymes, thus there may be a reduction in the total number of receptors available within that cell. This process is sometimes called receptor down-regulation, and is a common response of a receptor population to continued, excessive stimulation, this is one basis of drug tolerance (see later).

Another form of drug tolerance involves a reduction in the number of receptors available following a reduction of receptor synthesis, this takes somewhat longer to occur than the invagination desribed above. Again, this form of down-regulation may occur following repeated stimulation of the receptor by its agonist, or as a result of stimulation of another receptor, in which case it is called heterologous down-regulation. An increase in receptor synthesis may produce up-regulation.

In some cases, the responses to the circulating drug may decrease without there being any change in the number of receptors available. This is a rapid response and is called receptor desensitisation. There are various mechanisms by which this may be achieved, including a change in the affinity of the receptor for its drug, which may indicate a slight change in the chemical structure of the receptor or a decrease in the ability of the receptor to cause the synthesis of its second messenger, such effects are usually the result of phosphorylation of the receptor protein by enzymes such as receptor kinases, protein kinase C or cAMP-dependent kinases. These kinases usually have greatest affinity for the receptor when it is coupled to its agonist, hence the chain of events would be: the agonist–receptor interaction, resulting in synthesis of a second messenger which stimulates protein kinases; the protein kinases then, amongst other things, regulate the ability of the receptor to stimulate the G-protein, thus exerting a form of negative feedback control on receptor activity.

Receptor stimulation results in activation of protein kinases which may phosphorylate the receptor protein itself: a form of negative feedback

The importance of an appreciation of the possibility of a change in receptor activity is that there are some disorders where there are clinical symptoms of either chemical messenger excess or deficiency in the presence of normal circulating concentrations of that messenger. In these cases the cause of the disorder lies at the receptor level rather than at the messenger level.

■ SUMMARY

- Drugs may be defined as chemicals that cause a change in the normal activity of the body; responses to drug action may be classified as either graded, where the response can increase in magnitude, or quantal, where the response is 'all or nothing'. The effect of any drug is dependent upon the dose used, thus an increase in dose induces an increase in response in the case of graded responses or, in the case of quantal responses, an increase in the proportion of the population exhibiting the response. The dose–response relationship is not linear, the effect of the drug reaches a maximum at higher doses, after which an increase in dose does not cause an increase in response. It is common to portray the relationship between dose and response using a graph of the response versus the logarithm of the dose (or drug concentration), this not only allows a wider range of doses to be plotted, but also gives a curve, the central portion of which is approximately linear.

- The nature of the dose–response relationship can be explained using the 'lock and key' hypothesis of receptors. An increase in drug concentration results in a greater number of drug–receptor interactions and thus a greater response; occupation of all available receptors results in the maximal response being achieved. The 'lock and key' hypothesis, however, must be modified to take into account the concepts of affinity, intrinsic activity and spare receptors.

- One group of drugs has affinity for the receptor, but lacks intrinsic activity. These drugs, antagonists, interact with the receptors but do not produce an effect, other than to prevent access to the receptor by full agonists. Thus antagonists reduce the effects of agonists. Antagonists may be either competitive, in which case they bind to the same sites on the receptor as the agonists, or they may be non-competitive, in which case they bind to separate, but closely associated sites.

- The molecular nature of receptors is now well understood. Some receptors are intracellular and act by influencing intracellular enzyme activity or gene expression/transcription and protein synthesis. Because of the mechanism of action, drugs acting on these receptors are often slow in onset of action, but long in duration. The largest group of receptors are membrane bound, thus the drug does not need to enter the cell to influence cellular activity. Membrane-bound receptors may be associated with carrier proteins and ion channels, where the effect of the drug is to either increase or decrease movement of chemicals or ions to or from the cytoplasm. Drugs acting via these receptors usually elicit rapid responses. Another group of membrane-bound receptors are the membrane-bound enzymes, such as tyrosine kinase; activation of these receptors causes a chain of events resulting in cell differentiation and proliferation. Drugs acting on these receptors therefore have long-lasting effects. The final type of receptors are the G-protein coupled receptors. Activation of these receptors results in the modulation of ion channel activity or second messenger production. The second messengers then influence the activity of intracellular enzymes, resulting in rapid cellular responses. The involvement of G-proteins in receptor activity is important because it allows some degree of intracellular co-ordination of the activity of multiple receptors, it also explains the phenomenon of spare receptors.

- Receptor populations are dynamic, they are able to change in response to changes in the surrounding internal environment. Receptor disorders, some of them genetic, are involved in the aetiology of several diseases.

■ REVISION QUESTIONS

For each question select the most appropriate answer. Correct answers are presented in Appendix 1.

1. The maximal response:
   (a) is usually death;
   (b) is the response elicited by a dose equivalent to twice the ED_{50};
   (c) is obtained when all of the available receptors have been occupied;
   (d) is that response obtained when an increase in dose produces no increase in response;
   (e) is that response obtained when it is no longer possible to increase the dose.

2. Antagonists are drugs which:
   (a) bind to the same sites as the agonists;
   (b) have greater affinity for the receptor than agonists;
   (c) bind to the agonist to reduce its effects;
   (d) bind to the receptor to reduce the actions of the agonist;
   (e) bind to the receptor to produce effects opposite to those produced by the agonist.

3. Some drugs utilise membrane-bound receptors to elicit their response because:
   (a) membrane-bound receptors induce rapid effects;
   (b) membrane-bound receptors induce large effects;
   (c) the drug does not need to cross the blood vessel wall to produce its effects;
   (d) the drug does not need to cross the target cell wall to produce its effects;
   (e) membrane-bound receptors always produce consistent responses.

4. Examples of important second messengers involved in hormone actions are:
   (a) cAMP, IL-2, GST;
   (b) IP_3, cAMP, cGMP;
   (c) GAD, IP_3, GTP;

(d)   DAG, ATP, PO_3;

(e)   cAMP, DNA, ATP.

5.   G-protein coupled receptors:

(a)   all induce an increase in intracellular cAMP when stimulated;

(b)   all produce responses which are slow in onset, but very long lasting;

(c)   all have similar 'seven transmembrane domain' structures;

(d)   all utilise second messengers;

(e)   all act independently of ligand-gated ion channels.

6.   Which of the following is *not* true about tyrosine kinase receptors:

(a)   tyrosine kinase receptors are single-chain transmembrane proteins, which may dimerise;

(b)   tyrosine kinase receptors may phosphorylate the receptor protein itself;

(c)   tyrosine kinase receptors influence cell differentiation and replication by interacting directly with DNA;

(d)   tyrosine kinase receptors influence cell differentiation and replication by influencing MAP kinase (MAPK);

(e)   many hormones act via tyrosine kinase receptors.

■ SELECTED READING

Brody, T.M. and Garrison, J.C. (1998) Sites of action: receptors. In Brody, T.M., Larner, J. and Minneman, K.P. (eds) *Human Pharmacology: Molecular to Clinical* (Third edition), (St. Louis: Mosby), 9–25.

Garrison, J.C. (1998) Hormone receptors and signaling mechanisms. In Brody, T.M., Larner, J. and Minneman, K.P. (eds) *Human Pharmacology: Molecular to Clinical* (Third edition), (St. Louis: Mosby), 471–484.

Rang, H.P., Dale, M.M. and Ritter, J.M. (1999) How drugs act: molecular aspects. In Rang, H.P., Dale, M.M. and Ritter, J.M. *Pharmacology* (Fourth edition), (Edinburgh: Churchill Livingstone), 19–46.

Ross, E.M. (1996) Pharmacodynamics: mechanisms of drug action and the relationship between drug concentration and effect. In Hardman, J.G., Linbird, L.E. and Gilman, A.G. (eds) *Goodman and Gilman's The pharmacological basis of therapeutics* (Ninth edition), (New York: McGraw-Hill), 24–41.

■ COMPUTER-AIDED LEARNING PACKAGES

Further details of these learning packages can be found at
http://cbl.leeds.ac.uk/raven/pha/phCAL.html

Drug Targets and Transduction Mechanisms (version 1.96), Pharma-CAL-ogy, British Pharmacological Society, University of Leeds.

Introduction and How Receptors are Made and Regulated, Pharma-CAL-ogy, British Pharmacological Society, University of Leeds.

Enzymes as Drug Targets, Pharma-CAL-ogy, British Pharmacological Society, University of Leeds.

Steroid Receptors as Drug Targets, Pharma-CAL-ogy, British Pharmacological Society, University of Leeds.

Uptake and Transporter Systems as Drug Targets, Pharma-CAL-ogy, British Pharmacological Society, University of Leeds.

Tyrosine Kinase Receptors as Drug Targets, Pharma-CAL-ogy, British Pharmacological Society, University of Leeds.

G-Protein Receptors as Drug Targets, Pharma-CAL-ogy, British Pharmacological Society, University of Leeds.

Ion Channel Receptors as Drug Targets, Pharma-CAL-ogy, British Pharmacological Society, University of Leeds.

DRUGS ACTING ON THE PERIPHERAL NERVOUS SYSTEM

■ 2.1 INTRODUCTION

The human body is able to function in a variety of environments and in various conditions, for example it can adapt to changes in temperature and can cope with changes in nutritional status (e.g. fasting). The two control systems that enable this adaptation are the nervous system and the endocrine system. The nervous system is able to respond rapidly to changes in temperature or to threat or to injury, whereas the endocrine system is much slower to respond, and is therefore more concerned with long-term changes such as growth and reproduction. Disorders of either of these systems results in illness, which in some cases may be fatal. Both systems are also important in controlling the body's response to illness or injury and are therefore involved in the manifestation of the symptoms of disease. An understanding of the physiology of the endocrine and nervous systems has enabled the development of a myriad of drugs which are of use in the treatment of a wide range of illnesses, or which may be used to relieve the symptoms of disease. This chapter will discuss some aspects of drug action on the nervous system, drugs which influence the endocrine system are described in Chapter 8. The use of the drugs which influence the peripheral nervous system for the relief of disorders of the cardiovascular, respiratory or gastrointestinal sytems, for example, is described in more detail in the relevant chapters of this text.

■ 2.2 THE ANATOMY OF THE PERIPHERAL NERVOUS SYSTEM

The nervous system is divided into the central nervous system and the peripheral nervous system. The central nervous system, which is comprised of the brain and the spinal cord, is responsible for controlling the activity of the peripheral nervous system and is the seat of the higher mental functions, such as emotion, memory and learning. The central nervous system also plays an important role in controlling the endocrine system. Disorders of the central nervous system and the effects of drugs on brain and spinal function are described in Chapter 3.

The peripheral nervous system is divided into the autonomic and the somatic systems. The somatic nervous system is that part of the peripheral nervous system involved with the conduction of sensory information, such as touch, heat and pain, from the periphery to the brain and the conduction of nerve impulses from the brain to the skeletal muscles.

The somatic nervous system is concerned with sensory input and motor control of skeletal muscles, i.e. conscious actions

The important aspect of the somatic nervous system is that it is concerned with voluntary or conscious actions, for example eating or walking, although some of its activity is under reflex control, which means that it happens without deliberate intention, for example coughing. An important feature of these somatic reflexes is that they can be inhibited consciously, for example it is possible to suppress the cough reflex. Nerves that carry information to the central nervous system from the periphery are called afferent nerves, those that carry information from the brain to the effector organ or tissue, for example skeletal muscle, are called efferent nerves.

The autonomic nervous system is concerned with involuntary activity, it controls the body's vital functions. It is the autonomic nervous system that controls body temperature, blood pressure, respiration rate, etc., these processes are constantly being modified, usually without the individual being aware of the changes that are occurring, nor the reasons why. The autonomic nervous system is also comprised of afferent and efferent nerves: the afferent nerves carry the information from the various sensors, such as those which monitor blood pressure, to the brain; the efferent nerves then conduct the nerve impulses from the brain to the organs or tissues responsible for eliciting the response. In general terms, those areas of the brain concerned with autonomic function are the 'lower' areas such as the brainstem and midbrain, the areas concerned with voluntary, conscious activity are the 'higher' areas such as the cerebrocortex.

The efferent portion of the autonomic nervous system is further divided into the sympathetic nervous system and the parasympathetic nervous system. The sympathetic nervous system can be thought of as being that part of the autonomic nervous system that is concerned with the response to stressful or threatening events in the environment. At times of stress it is the sympathetic nervous system that causes the increase in rate and force of contraction of the heart, that directs the blood flow towards the skeletal muscle and away from the skin and the gut, and that liberates carbohydrates from stores. All of these actions permit the body to respond to the stress or threat effectively and rapidly. The parasympathetic nervous system generally acts in a way opposite to the sympathetic nervous system and is more concerned with body function at times of rest and calm, thus it decreases heart rate and increases the secretory and motile activity of the gastrointestinal tract.

The divisions of the peripheral nervous system are illustrated in figure 2.1. As well as there being functional differences between the various divisions of the peripheral

The autonomic nervous system controls unconscious, involuntary functions such as heart rate and gastrointestinal activity

The sympathetic nervous system is important when the body is active, the parasympathetic when the body is at rest

• **Figure 2.1** The functional divisions of the peripheral nervous system

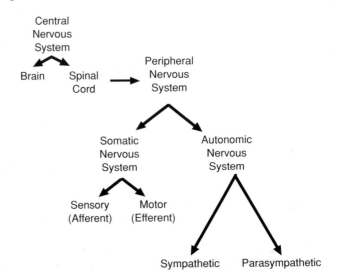

nervous system, there are also anatomical differences. The somatic nerves can be myelinated or unmyelinated, the afferent fibres normally travel from their receptors to the spinal cord where they synapse with a second fibre which then conducts the impulse to the brain. Similarly efferent impulses are conducted down the spinal cord where the fibres synapse with motor neurones which carry the impulse to the skeletal muscle. Neurones of the autonomic nervous system differ in that they leave the spinal cord and travel to a ganglion or 'relay centre'. In the case of the sympathetic nervous system the preganglionic nerve fibres leave the spinal cord in the thoracic and lumbar regions and then travel to ganglia which are situated in two single chains running a short distance from, and aligned with, the spinal column itself. These short preganglionic sympathetic nerve fibres are usually myelinated. The postganglionic sympathetic fibres then run from the ganglion to the effector organ or tissue, this distance may be quite large. Postganglionic sympathetic fibres are generally unmyelinated (see figure 2.2). In contrast, the ganglia of the para-sympathetic nervous system are usually within, or very close to, the effector organ. As with the sympathetic nervous system, the preganglionic fibre of the parasympathetic nerve is myelinated, and the postganglionic fibre is unmyelinated.

The somatic, sympathetic autonomic and parasympathetic autonomic systems also differ in the neurotransmitters and receptor subtypes used at the synapses of the ganglia and at the points at which the nerve meets its target muscle or gland, known as the neuroeffector junction. These differences, and the implications for drug action and therapeutics, will be discussed in Sections 2.4, 2.5 and 2.6. The other aspect of the nervous system that is amenable to moderation by drugs is the nerve action potential itself. The ability to prevent the conduction of a nerve impulse would allow the control of muscle or glandular activity by the central or autonomic nervous systems to be moderated and would allow sensory input such as pain to be inhibited. The actions and uses of drugs which interfere with the conduction of the nerve action potential are described in Section 2.3.

■ 2.3 DRUGS AFFECTING THE NERVE IMPULSE

As described in Chapter 1, Section 1.4.2.1, the nerve action potential is propagated by the opening of voltage-gated sodium channels, which allow the influx of sodium into the cell and the depolarisation of that cell, followed by the opening of voltage-gated potassium channels which allow efflux of potassium ions from the cell and therefore repolarisation of that cell. Blockade of the voltage-gated sodium channels prevents the depolarisation of the cell and therefore prevents the propagation of the action potential. Local anaesthetic agents act by binding to the sodium channel, some by binding at an intracellular site, thereby preventing the movement of sodium ions; because some of the drugs must first enter the cell for them to act, these drugs are more effective against open channels (i.e. active neurones) than resting channels. A list of common local anaesthetic agents is presented in Box 2.1.

Local anaesthetics act on all types of nerve, thus they prevent nerve conduction in the central and peripheral somatic and autonomic nerves, both afferent and efferent. It has been shown, however, that they are most effective against smaller diameter nerve fibres, and also against myelinated nerves. The reason for the greater effect against myelinated nerves is the need to act only at the nodes of Ranvier rather than across the whole nerve cell membrane. The extent of the local anaesthesia can be moderated by the choice of method of administration, for example surface, infiltration, nerve block, epidural or spinal. Surface anaesthesia is where the drug is applied directly to the surface that is to be anaesthetised, for example the cornea. Another form of surface anaesthesia is topical anaesthesia where the drug is applied to the skin in the form of a cream. Infiltration is

• **Figure 2.2** A schematic representation of the anatomical differences between the sympathetic and parasympathetic divisions of the autonomic nervous system

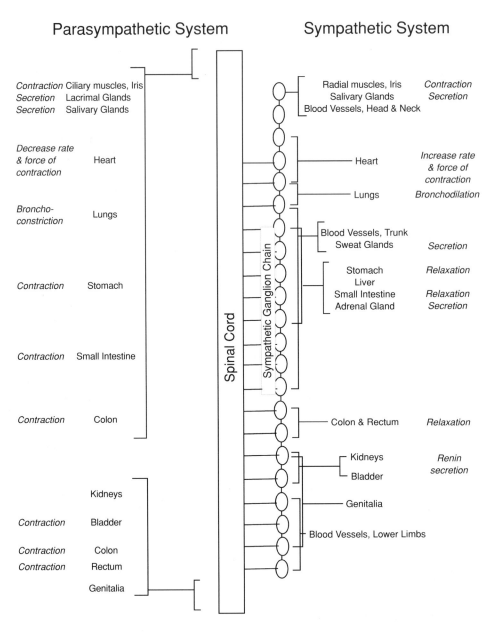

Parasympathetic System

Contraction Ciliary muscles, Iris
Secretion Lacrimal Glands
Secretion Salivary Glands

Decrease rate & force of contraction — Heart

Broncho-constriction — Lungs

Contraction — Stomach

Contraction — Small Intestine

Contraction — Colon

Kidneys
Contraction Bladder
Contraction Colon
Contraction Rectum
Genitalia

Sympathetic System

Spinal Cord

Sympathetic Ganglion Chain

Radial muscles, Iris — *Contraction*
Salivary Glands — *Secretion*
Blood Vessels, Head & Neck

Heart — *Increase rate & force of contraction*

Lungs — *Bronchodilation*

Blood Vessels, Trunk
Sweat Glands — *Secretion*

Stomach — *Relaxation*
Liver
Small Intestine — *Relaxation*
Adrenal Gland — *Secretion*

Colon & Rectum — *Relaxation*

Kidneys — *Renin secretion*
Bladder

Genitalia

Blood Vessels, Lower Limbs

where the drug is injected below the skin, usually at several sites close to the area to be anaesthetised, this allows anaesthesia to a deeper level than surface anaesthesia and therefore permits incision into, or excision of, the anaesthetised tissue. A nerve block is achieved by injecting the local anaesthetic close to a major nerve bundle, by doing this all nerve conduction to or from tissues distal to the nerve block are inhibited. This form of anaes-thesia is particularly useful in dental surgery and for surgery to limbs, where the whole limb can be anaesthetised by one single injection, for example to the shoulder or upper arm. Another form of nerve block, is the pudendal nerve block, used to relieve the pain of childbirth; the pudendal nerve innervates the genitalia.

Local anaesthetics block nerve conduction in all nerves, but they are only used therapeutically to block conduction in those nerves carrying the pain sensation

■ *Box 2.1* Commonly used local anaesthetic agents

Agent	Proprietary name	Uses
Amethocaine (tetracaine)	Amitop®	Surface anaesthesia
Benzocaine	Various	Throat lozenges
Bupivacaine	Marcain®	Epidural and spinal anaesthesia
Lignocaine (lidocaine)	Xylocaine®, Instillagel®	Surface and infiltration anaesthesia
Mepivacaine	Scandonest®	Dental anaesthesia
Prilocaine	Citanest®	Infiltration, regional and dental anaesthesia
Ropivacaine	Naropin®	Epidural anaesthesia

Spinal anaesthesia is achieved by injection of the local anaesthetic into the spinal canal; by doing this sensory and motor information coming from, or going to, the whole lower part of the body can be blocked. The extent of the block depends on the site of injection, thus anaesthesia in the lower spine anaesthetises a more limited area than anaesthesia of the spine in the cervical region. This form of anaesthesia can be complicated by the fact that the spinal canal is only easily accessible in certain areas, a problem that can be overcome by formulation of the anaesthetic so that it floats within the cerebrospinal fluid, thus anaesthetising an area above the site of injection, or formulating the drug so that it sinks. Epidural anaesthesia is where the anaesthetic is injected into the outer part of the spinal cord. The consequence of epidural anaesthesia is to prevent nerve impulses entering or leaving the spinal cord at the level of the site of injection, but without having any effect on the transmission of impulses within the cord itself, that is, impulses arising from areas below the site of injection. The benefit of epidural anaesthesia over spinal anaesthesia, for example during childbirth, is the ability to anaesthetise a defined area of the body, for example pelvic organs, without disrupting more distal tissues, such as the legs.

The site of administration of a local anaesthetic dictates its extent of activity, a single injection into the spine can anaesthetise the whole lower body

One of the important features of local anaesthetics is their safety and reversibility. The drugs are only effective while they are blocking the sodium channel, their efficacy is lost by diffusion away from the site of action. Once the drugs have diffused away from the nerves, nerve function is fully regained, and the drug is ineffective at any other non-neuronal site, with the possible exception of cardiac tissue (see Chapter 4). The various local anaesthetic drugs differ mainly in their duration of action, which is a function of their lipid solubility. Lipid-soluble drugs are less soluble in the aqueous blood and therefore diffuse away from the site of action more slowly. More lipid-soluble drugs therefore tend to have a greater duration of action. In some cases the anaesthetic is injected along with adrenaline (epinephrine). The adrenaline acts to constrict peripheral blood vessels and therefore to limit the diffusion of anaesthetic agent further, thereby extending the duration of action.

■ 2.4 NEUROMUSCULAR BLOCKERS

Neuromuscular blocking drugs are more selective than local anaesthetics, in that they only prevent transmission of the action potential at the point of interaction between a somatic efferent (motor) nerve and skeletal muscle; they have no effect on afferent nerves or on afferent nerves of the autonomic nervous system.

At the neuromuscular junction the terminal of the somatic nerve releases acetylcholine (ACh), this acetylcholine then reacts with cholinergic receptors of the nicotinic subtype, situated on the muscle fibre. Each muscle fibre is innervated by a single motor neurone, and the action of the acetylcholine is to cause the opening of ion channels, which results in an increased permeability to sodium, potassium and, to some extent, calcium ions; this causes muscle fibre depolarisation and ultimately muscle contraction. The acetylcholine is then broken down by acetylcholinesterase present at the neuromuscular junction, or by butyrylcholinesterase in the plasma. This process allows for repeated muscle contraction, or even tetany (sustained contraction), but persistent activation of the nicotinic receptors has the effect of causing the voltage-gated sodium ion channels to become refractory. In the refractory state the sodium ion channel fails to open in response to the acetylcholine and therefore muscle contraction is prevented. A longer-term effect of repeated nicotic receptor stimulation is receptor desensitisation, which again results in diminished muscle contraction.

There are two classes of neuromuscular blocking agent: non-depolarising and depolarising. The first identified non-depolarising neuromuscular blocking agent was curare, the agent used to poison arrows by South American hunters. This chemical blocks neuromuscular transmission, thereby preventing the escape of the hunted animal, but is poorly absorbed by the oral route, meaning that the captured animals was still usable as a source of food. Drugs with actions similar to that of curare include tubocurarine, pancuronium, vecuronium, atracurium and gallamine. These drugs all act as competitive antagonists of acetylcholine at the nicotinic receptor of the neuromuscular junction. The effect of these non-depolarising neuromuscular blockers is to cause paralysis, with the muscles of the eye being the first muscles to be affected and the thoracic muscles of respiration being the last affected before death (from asphyxia). Other effects of these drugs arise from effects at the nicotinic receptors of the autonomic ganglia, which result in abolition of activity of both the sympathetic and parasympathetic systems (see Sections 2.5 and 2.6). Following blockade of the somatic neuromuscular junction, muscle function is regained either by competitive displacement of the blocker by acetylcholine or following metabolism or excretion of the agent.

Depolarising neuromuscular blockers act by stimulating the nicotinic receptor to excess, resulting in loss of muscle function following the entry of the voltage-gated sodium ion channels to an inactive, refractory state (see above). The difference between this form of neuromuscular blockade and that of the non-depolarising agents is the possibility of fasciculation (muscle tremors) prior to the onset of paralysis when using depolarising agents. The most important depolarising neuromuscular blocking agents are decamethonium and suxamethonium, of which only the latter is used therapeutically. Suxamethonium, which is known as succinylcholine in the USA, is comprised of two acetylcholine molecules linked by the acetyl groups. Reversal of the brief depolarising blockade occurs following metabolism of the suxamethonium.

Neuromuscular blocking agents are used therapeutically to enable intubation of the trachea or to relax muscles prior to surgery. The predominant problems with their use arise from paralysis of the respiratory muscles, which necessitates mechanical ventilation, and the fact that they do not suppress consciousness nor the pain sensation, but they do prevent the ability to respond to pain, for example twitch or speak. In therapeutic use the effects of the non-depolarising agents can be reversed by the administration of an inhibitor of cholinesterase, this has the effect of increasing the concentration of

Curare, a non-depolarising neuromuscular blocker, is used in South America for the poisoning of arrows for hunting

■ *Box 2.2* The aetiology and treatment of myaesthenia gravis

Myasthenia gravis is a condition that affects approximately 0.05% of the population. It is characterised by extreme muscle weakness and fatigue, particularly after repeated muscle contraction. One particular feature of myasthenia gravis is 'drooping eyelids' because the muscles concerned with blinking are used repetitively, but unconsciously; the muscle fatigue and weakness is therefore manifested here before being manifested in other skeletal muscles. The cause of myasthenia gravis is a decrease in the number of nicotinic cholinergic receptors at the neuromuscular junction, there sometimes being up to 70% loss of receptors. This receptor destruction is due to an autoimmune disorder which results in the production of antibodies to the acetylcholine receptors of the neuromuscular junction, other receptor subtypes are unaffected. Treatment of myasthenia gravis involves administration of inhibitors of cholinesterase, this has the effect of increasing the functional 'life span' of any released acetylcholine, which is then able to stimulate those receptors that are still available.

Sadly, as the disease progresses the number of available nicotinic receptors decreases, and the beneficial effect of the enzyme inhibitor declines. In such cases, an alternative approach to treatment is the prevention of antibody formation, for example by the administration of corticosteroids (see Chapter 9).

acetylcholine at the neuromuscular junction which displaces the antagonists from the receptors; anticholinesterases potentiate the effects of the depolarising agents by enhancing the already excessive receptor stimulation. Inhibitors of cholinesterase can also be used in the treatment of myasthenia gravis (see Box 2.2).

Other mechanisms by which neuromuscular transmission can be prevented are the inhibition of acetylcholine synthesis in the nerve terminal or by inhibition of acetylcholine release. Hemicholinium acts to inhibit choline uptake into the nerve terminal, this has the effect of preventing acetylcholine synthesis, and therefore neuromuscular transmission, but the lack of specificity of the effect means that the drug cannot be used therapeutically because it also prevents acetylcholine synthesis within neurones of the autonomic nervous system. Acetylcholine release is inhibited by the toxin of *Clostridium botulinum* (botulinum toxin), this effect explains the extreme toxicity of this toxin, but also renders it useful as a muscle relaxant to relieve muscle spasticity when injected locally into the muscle. β-Bungarotoxin, a component of cobra venom, also inhibits acetylcholine release, thus causing paralysis of the victim.

■ 2.5 DRUGS ACTING ON THE SYMPATHETIC NERVOUS SYSTEM

As described in Section 2.2, the myelinated nerves of the sympathetic nervous system leave the spinal cord and travel the short distance to the chain of sympathetic ganglia that lies alongside the spinal cord. At the ganglia these preganglionic fibres synapse with postganglionic fibres, which then conduct the impulse to the effector organ or tissue. Sympathetic, postganglionic fibres are non-myelinated. The neurotransmitter utilised within the ganglia is acetylcholine, which acts on cholinergic nicotinic receptors; these ganglionic nicotinic receptors are different from those found at the neuromuscular junction (Section 2.4). The neurotransmitter released at the neuroeffector junction of the sympathetic nervous system is noradrenaline, which in the USA is called norepinephrine. The released noradrenaline acts on adrenoceptors, of which there are several subtypes: α_1; α_2; β_1; β_2 and β_3.

In the sympathetic nervous system the noradrenaline acts on adrenoceptors, of which there are several subtypes: α_1; α_2; β_1; β_2 and β_3

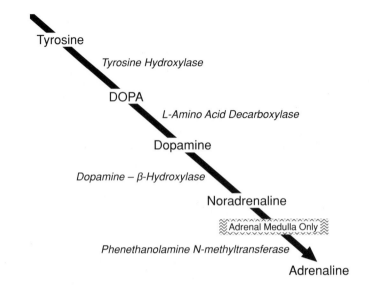

• Figure 2.3 The synthetic pathway for the production of noradrenaline and adrenaline from tyrosine

Tyrosine

Tyrosine Hydroxylase

DOPA

L-Amino Acid Decarboxylase

Dopamine

Dopamine – β-Hydroxylase

Noradrenaline

Adrenal Medulla Only

Phenethanolamine N-methyltransferase

Adrenaline

Within the ganglia the acetylcholine is synthesised in the same way as it is in the neuromuscular junction: by the acetylation of choline by choline acetyltransferase, using acetyl coenzyme A as the acetyl donor; again metabolism of acetylcholine is by acetylcholinesterase. At the neuroeffector junction, noradrenaline is synthesised from the amino acid tyrosine via dopamine (see figure 2.3), using the same synthetic pathway as is used in the brain (Chapter 3) and in the medulla of the adrenal gland (Chapter 8). Deactivation of the noradrenaline occurs by several processes, the first is a reuptake process, called uptake$_1$, in which the noradrenaline is taken back up into the prejunctional terminal for re-use. There is also an uptake$_2$ process, where the transmitter is taken up into the postjunctional cell for metabolism by catechol-O-methyl transferase (COMT). The final means of deactivation of noradrenaline is by monoamine oxidase (MAO) which is present in mitochondria.

Each of the adrenoceptors on which the noradrenaline acts has a different function, thus they are distributed at different sites around the body and utilise various second messenger sytems. α_1-Adrenoceptors are found predominantly in blood vessels and in the smooth muscles of the genitourinary system. These seven transmembrane domain G-protein coupled receptors are linked to G_q, which causes the production of diacylglycerol and inositol triphosphate, the ultimate effect of which is to cause smooth muscle contraction. The α_2-adrenoceptors are found in some blood vessels and in the gastrointestinal tract; they are also present in the pancreas and on blood platelets. α_2-Adrenoceptors are linked to G_i and therefore they cause a decrease in cyclic AMP synthesis, which results in contraction of smooth muscle, platelet aggregation and decrease in secretion of insulin. Most α_2-adrenoceptors, however, are presynaptic, where they function as autoreceptors to decrease the release of noradrenaline at the sympathetic neuroeffector junction.

All three subtypes of the β-adrenoceptors are linked to G_s; they therefore stimulate adenylyl cyclase to cause synthesis of cyclic AMP. β_1-Adrenoceptors are found predominantly in the heart, where they cause an increase in the rate and force of contraction. They are also found in the kidney, where they influence renin release (see Chapter 4), and on adipocytes where they induce lipolysis. The β_2-adrenoceptors are found in the lung, where they cause bronchodilation and in the blood vessels which supply skeletal muscle, where they cause vasodilation. β_3-Adrenoceptors are associated with adipocytes, where they have a role similar to that of the β_1-adrenoceptors.

Drugs are able to influence the activity of the sympathetic nervous system by several means, for example they can mimic the transmitter, they can block the actions of the transmitter or they can prevent transmitter inactivation. The predominant effect of any such drug would depend on the adrenoceptor subtypes affected. Drugs which act directly on the adrenoceptors are called direct-acting sympathomimetics, these are classical agonists of the receptors. Noradrenaline and adrenaline are able to stimulate all types of adrenoceptors, although their relative efficacies differ: noradrenaline has a predominantly α-adrenoceptor effect, unlike adrenaline which is equally effective at stimulating the α- and β-adrenoceptors. For therapeutic use, drugs with more selective actions are of greatest benefit because they are less likely to cause unwanted ('side') effects. Examples of such agents are phenylephrine and methoxamine, which are selective agonists of α_1-adrenoceptors. These drugs are administered locally to the nose to induce vasoconstriction, they are therefore useful as decongestants. If they were to be given systemically, the widespread vasoconstriction would induce an increase in blood pressure followed by a reflex decrease in the rate and force of contraction of the heart (see Chapter 4). There are also selective agonists of α_2-adrenoceptors, but none of these are used therapeutically; clonidine, an α_2-adrenoceptor agonist with some α_1-adrenoceptor agonist properties is used in the treatment of migraine, menopausal hot flushes and hypertension, but these uses may owe more to effects on central (brain) α-adrenoceptors than on peripheral receptors.

Agonists of α-adrenoceptors are used as decongestants whereas agonists of β-adrenoceptors are used to treat heart failure and asthma

Isoprenaline (known in the USA as isoproterenol), is an agonist at β_1- and β_2-adrenoceptors. When administered systemically this drug dilates bronchial smooth muscle, and can therefore be of use in the treatment of disorders such as asthma (see Chapter 6), but it also causes dilation of blood vessels supplying skeletal muscle, the result of which is a decrease in blood pressure. As a reflex response to the decrease in blood pressure there is an increase in the rate and force of contraction of the heart, an effect enhanced by the effects of the isoprenaline on the β_1-adrenoceptors of the heart; the use of isoprenaline for the relief of asthma is therefore accompanied by cardiac symptoms such as tachycardia. One method by which these side-effects can be decreased is by administration of the drug locally to the lungs, for example by use of an inhaler, but there may still be cardiac effects. The other method by which sympathomimetics can be used to relieve asthma without inducing cardiac effects is to use selective agonists of the β_2-adrenoceptors, such as salbutamol (which in the USA is called albuterol). Salbutamol is able to induce bronchodilation without inducing cardiac effects, although it is usual to give the drug by inhalation to decrease the risk of peripheral vasodilation and the sequelae of the induced hypotension. It should not be thought, however, that stimulation of the heart via β_1-adrenoceptors is of no therapeutic use. In cases of heart failure it is possible to increase the activity of the heart by administration of adrenaline, such actions are beneficial but there are associated risks arising from the other effects of this catecholamine, for example peripheral vasoconstriction via an effect on α_1-adrenoceptors. Dobutamine is a selective agonist of β_1-adrenoceptors used to stimulate activity of the heart without inducing effects on α- or β_2-adrenoceptors, it is therefore safer to use this for the relief of heart failure than adrenaline.

Another group of sympathomimetics are the indirect-acting sympathomimetics, which act by inducing the release of noradrenaline from the neuroeffector junction, or by preventing the inactivation of noradrenaline. Examples of such drugs are tyramine, ephedrine, pseudoephedrine and amphetamine (amfetamine), and the monoamine oxidase inhibitors such as tranylcypromine. These drugs are important because they also induce noradrenaline release, or prevent noradrenaline inactivation, in the central nervous system, and therefore act as psychostimulants (see Chapter 3), but their effects in the periphery are limited. The most important peripheral effect of these drugs is the potential to induce hypertension due to the predominant effect on the α_1-adrenoceptors, this is the basis of the 'cheese effect' of tyramine in users of monoamine oxidase inhibitors (see Chapter 3, Section 3.3.1).

Another way in which the actions of the sympathetic nervous system can be influenced by drugs is by antagonism of the adrenoceptors. Again, the type of effect caused depends on the selectivity or the adrenoceptor antagonist. There are several antagonists of α-adrenoceptors: phenoxybenzamine and phentolamine are non-selective antagonists of both α_1- and α_2-adrenoceptors, whereas prazosin and terazosin are selective antagonists of α_1-adrenoceptors; idazoxan is a selective α_2-adrenoceptor antagonist. Administration of these agents causes inhibition of vasoconstriction, i.e. vasodilation. This has the effect of lowering blood pressure. In many cases the decreased blood pressure is accompanied by a reflex increase in heart rate. This reflex tachycardia, however, is less for selective α_1-adrenoceptor agonists because the α_2-adrenoceptors are unaffected and therefore still able to moderate noradrenaline release. α-Adrenoceptor antagonists also inhibit the noradrenaline-induced contractions of smooth muscle in the genitourinary tract and can therefore be used to relieve the urinary retention of benign prostate hyperplasia, although another effect of these agents is inhibition of ejaculation due to effects on the vas deferens.

β-Adrenoceptor antagonists are of greater therapeutic use than α-adrenoceptor antagonists. Antagonism of β_1-adrenoceptors causes a decrease in the rate and force of contraction of the heart, this effect is of great importance in the treatment of angina and hypertension (see Chapter 4). The archetypal β-adrenoceptor antagonist is propranolol, which has been used for several decades. However, propranolol is a non-selective β_1- and β_2-adrenoceptor antagonist. Use of this agent is therefore accompanied by effects on the arterioles supplying skeletal muscle and on adipocytes, although these adverse effects are rarely troublesome because of the presence of other compensatory mechanisms. Clinically, the most important adverse effect of propranolol is the effects on the lungs, where it prevents the bronchodilatory effects of endogenous noradrenaline and therefore causes bronchoconstriction, giving rise to the symptoms of asthma. This adverse effect of propranolol has been reduced by the development of selective β_1-adrenoceptor antagonists, such as atenolol and metoprolol, which are effective in the treatment of hypertension and angina, but have few effects on the lung, although their use by asthmatics is still not recommended. There are no clinical indications for the development of a selective β_2-adrenoceptor antagonist, which would be expected to cause bronchoconstriction, decreased blood flow to skeletal muscle and therefore increased peripheral resistance.

The activity of the sympathetic nervous system can also be decreased by inhibition of noradrenaline release at the neuroeffector junction. This can be achieved by use of drugs such as guanethidine, which prevents noradrenaline release in response to an action potential or an indirectly acting sympathomimetic; reserpine prevents storage of noradrenaline in the nerve terminal. These drugs are all useful in the treatment of hypertension, but because of the non-selectivity of their action, their use is often accompanied by side-effects such as increased gut motility and diarrhoea and effects on the genitourinary system; it is because of these effects that these drugs are only used as a 'last resort', preference being given to the more selective agents such as atenolol.

A final way in which the activity of the sympathetic nervous system can be decreased is by blocking the actions of the acetylcholine at the ganglion. Such an effect can be achieved

Propranolol is used to treat hypertension and angina but also causes the predictable side-effect of asthma

by use of the nicotinic antagonists hexamethonium or trimetaphan. These drugs reduce sympathetic activity and could therefore be used to decrease blood pressure, but because the parasympathetic nervous system also uses acetylcholine as the transmitter at the ganglia, these drugs also reduce parasympathetic nervous system activity. The net effect of ganglion blocker use therefore depends on which effect is normally dominant; thus in the heart, where the parasympathetic effect is normally dominant, ganglion blockers would cause tachycardia, whereas in the vasculature, which has no parasympathetic input, ganglion blockers would cause general vasodilation. It is because of the unpredictability of these effects that ganglion blockers are only rarely used in therapeutics. As mentioned in Section 2.4 above, non-depolarising neuromuscular blocking agents also have some effect on autonomic ganglia, preventing ganglionic transmission. The use of neuromuscular blocking agents may therefore be accompanied by effects similar to those seen with hexamethonium or trimetaphan.

■ 2.6 DRUGS ACTING ON THE PARASYMPATHETIC NERVOUS SYSTEM

The parasympathetic nervous system has many similarities with the sympathetic nervous system, but also many differences. Like the sympathetic nervous system, the preganglionic nerve fibre of the parasympathetic system is myelinated, and the postganglionic fibre non-myelinated, but in contrast to the sympathetic system, in the parasympathetic nervous system the preganglionic fibre is long, with the ganglion being adjacent to, or within the effector organ or tissue, and the postganglionic fibre is very short. Both nervous systems use acetylcholine as the transmitter within the ganglia, the acetylcholine acting on nicotinic receptors within the ganglia in both systems. In the parasympathetic nervous system, however, unlike the sympathetic nervous system, the transmitter at the neuroeffector junction is again acetylcholine, but in this case it acts on muscarinic receptors.

There are several subtypes of muscarinic receptor, named M_1 to M_5. In terms of the actions of the parasympathetic nervous system, the M_2 and M_3 receptors, which are found in the heart and in glands and smooth muscle respectively, are the most important. M_1 receptors are found in the ganglia, where they moderate the cholinergic transmission; the roles of M_4 and M_5 are poorly understood. M_1, M_2 and M_3 receptors are all coupled to G_q and therefore all utilise diacylglycerol and inositol triphosphate as second messengers.

As with the sympathetic nervous system, where there are direct-acting and indirect-acting sympathomimetics, there are also direct-acting and indirect-acting parasympathomimetics. Direct-acting parasympathomimetics include acetylcholine itself, carbachol and pilocarpine. Systemic administration of these agents would be expected to cause a decrease in heart rate, bronchoconstriction, contraction of the gastrointestinal tract, uterus and bladder, and constriction of the ciliary muscles of the eye. Because of these wide-ranging effects, and the lack of selective agonists of the various muscarinic receptor subtypes, these agents are not used systemically for any therapeutic purpose. They are, however, used for local administration to the eye to cause contraction of the muscles, which is of use in the relief of glaucoma (increased intraocular pressure). The only indirectly acting parasympathomimetics of consequence are ganglionic stimulants and inhibitors of acetylcholinesterase. These drugs act to potentiate the actions of acetylcholine but are not selective in the muscarinic or nicotinic effects, they therefore stimulate both the parasympathetic and sympathetic nervous systems. The clinical use of anticholinesterases for the reversal of neuromuscular blockade and the treatment of myasthenia gravis is described in Section 2.4. Another aspect of anticholinesterases are the irreversible anti-cholinesterase organophosphates that are used as insecticides and have been used in chemical

Organophosphates, the insecticides and chemical warfare agents, are irreversible inhibitors of cholinesterase

Muscarinic antagonists relieve asthma, but can also cause blurred vision, constipation and urinary retention

warfare. The effects of low-dose cholinesterase inhibition by organophosphates are limited to the neuromuscular junction, where there is increased force of contraction of skeletal muscles, but as the dose increases depolarising neuromuscular blockade ensues, causing paralysis (see Section 2.4). It is only at the higher doses that the autonomic effects become apparent, with the parasympathetic effects predominating, for example decreased heart rate and increased gut motility. At very high doses the effect at the sympathetic ganglia become apparent, with induction of increased rate and force of contraction of the heart.

Therapeutically, the most important group of drugs to act on the parasympathetic nervous system are the muscarinic antagonists such as atropine and scopolamine. Because of the lack of selectivity for subtypes of muscarinic receptors, these agents are effective in reducing the effects of all aspects of the parasympathetic nervous system. Administration of a muscarinic antagonist has the effect of relaxing non-vascular smooth muscle such as the gut and the lung, which can be of use in the relief of diarrhoea and asthma (see Chapters 7 and 6, respectively), but there are also effects on the bladder, which cause urinary retention, and on the heart, where they induce tachycardia. Effects on the central nervous system also result in sedation, which is sometimes used deliberately, for example in the prevention of motion sickness (see Chapter 7). The most important aspect of antimuscarinic actions is the association with drugs of many different classes, for example antipsychotic agents and antidepressant agents (see Chapter 3) and antihistamines (see Chapter 9). Many drugs in these groups exhibit marked antimuscarinic effects, and therefore produce the classical anticholinergic side-effects of blurred vision, dry mouth, constipation, urinary retention and sedation; all of these effects, and others, can be predicted from a knowledge of the actions of the parasympathetic nervous system.

As described above, in Section 2.5, it is also possible to reduce activity of the parasympathetic nervous system by antagonism of the nicotinic receptors of the ganglia. This approach, however, is of little therapeutic benefit because of the fact that the sympathetic nervous system utilises the same ganglionic transmission process and therefore such drugs have unpredictable effects, dependent on the dominance of either the sympathetic or parasympathetic systems.

■ SUMMARY

- The nervous system is divided into the central nervous system and the peripheral nervous system. The peripheral nervous system is then further divided into the somatic nervous system, which is concerned with sensation and motor control of skeletal muscle, and the autonomic nervous system, which is concerned with involuntary functions such as control of heart rate and gut motility. The autonomic nervous system is then further divided into the sympathetic and parasympathetic nervous systems. The sympathetic nervous system dominates when the body is active, thus it causes increased heart and respiration rate, whereas the parasympathetic system is concerned with rest, for example decreased heart rate and increased gastrointestinal motility.
- Disorders of the peripheral nervous system can cause severe illness but, more importantly, these systems are involved in the symptoms, for example pain, and treatment of many conditions.
- One class of drugs that inhibit the actions of the peripheral nervous system is the local anaesthetics. These drugs block the sodium ion channels of nerves and therefore prevent conduction of the action potential, but they are non-selective and therefore block conduction in both sensory and motor nerves and in nerves of the autonomic

nervous system. Local anaesthetics are used solely for the inhibition of pain, the extent of their activity being controlled by the site and method of administration.

- Neuomuscular blocking drugs are more selective than local anaesthetics, in that they only prevent transmission at the junction of the somatic motor nerve and the skeletal muscle. Neuromuscular blockers act either by antagonism of the muscle nicotinic cholinergic receptor (non-depolarising neuromuscular blockers) or by excessive stimulation of the receptor, which induces a refractory state in the sodium ion channel (depolarising neuromuscular blocker). Neuromuscular blocking drugs are used to facilitate tracheal intubation and to induce muscle relaxation prior to and during surgery.
- The activity of the sympathetic nervous system can be controlled in several ways: stimulation of the neuroeffector receptors; induced release of transmitter; antagonism of the receptors; or prevention of transmitter release. The effects of drugs with such actions depends on the receptor subtypes affected. Agonists of α-adrenoceptors induce vasoconstriction and can therefore be used as nasal decongestants, whereas agonists of β-adrenoceptors cause increased cardiac function and bronchodilation, depending on the subtype of β-adrenoceptor affected. These latter drugs can therefore be used to relieve acute heart failure or acute asthma. Antagonists of α-adrenoceptors induce vasoconstriction and can therefore be used to decrease blood pressure, as can antagonists of β-adrenoceptors, although these drugs may also induce asthma.
- The activity of the parasympathetic nervous system can be controlled in ways similar to those outlined for the sympathetic nervous system. Muscarinic cholinergic agonists are of little therapeutic use, with the exceptions of the treatment of glaucoma, but antagonists can be used to decrease heart rate, induce bronchodilation and decrease gastrointestinal motility. An appreciation of the actions of the parasympathetic nervous system is important for an understanding of the anticholinergic side-effects induced by many therapeutic agents.

■ REVISION QUESTIONS

For each question select the most appropriate answer. Correct answers are presented in Appendix 1.

1. Which of the following properties is *not* true for the parasympathetic nervous system:
   (a) the neurotransmitter at the ganglion is acetylcholine;
   (b) the neurotransmitter at the neuroeffector junction is acetylcholine;
   (c) the neurotransmitter at the neuroeffector junction is noradrenaline;
   (d) the receptors at the ganglion are cholinergic nicotinic;
   (e) the ganglia are situated close to the target organ.

2. Local anaesthetics act by blocking which of the following:
   (a) sodium–potassium ATPase;
   (b) chemically gated sodium ion channels;
   (c) chemically gated calcium ion channels;
   (d) voltage-gated sodium ion channels;
   (e) voltage-gated potassium ion channels.

3. Which of the following is *not* a form of local anaesthesia:
   (a) infiltration;
   (b) regional;
   (c) epidural;

    (d) spinal;

    (e) central.

4. Which of the following are true of the neuromuscular blocking agent suxamethonium:

    (a) suxamethonium is an antagonist of cholinergic nicotinic receptors at the neuromuscular junction;

    (b) suxamethonium stimulates cholinergic nicotinic receptors at the neuromuscular junction;

    (c) suxamethonium also prevents the pain sensation and can therefore be used as an anaesthetic;

    (d) suxamethonium is chemically related to nicotine;

    (e) suxamethonium was used by South Americans to aid hunting.

5. Which of the following are true of β_1-adrenoceptors:

    (a) β_1-adrenoceptors are found predominantly in the heart;

    (b) β_1-adrenoceptors are coupled to calcium ion channels;

    (c) β_1-adrenoceptors are predominantly presynaptic;

    (d) β_1-adrenoceptors act via the G_q subtype of G-protein;

    (e) antagonists of β_1-adrenoceptors increase the rate and force of contraction of the heart.

6. Organophosphate insecticides are:

    (a) antagonists of cholinergic nicotinic receptors;

    (b) antagonists of cholinergic muscarinic receptors;

    (c) directly acting sympathomimetics;

    (d) irreversible inhibitors of cholinesterase;

    (e) irreversible inhibitors of choline acetyltransferase.

■ SELECTED READING

Atchison, W.D. (1998) Neuromuscular blocking agents. In Brody, T.M., Larner, J. and Minneman, K.P. (eds) *Human Pharmacology: Molecular to Clinical* (Third edition), (St. Louis: Mosby), 143–150.

Bylund, D.B. (1998) Physiology and biochemistry of the peripheral autonomic nervous system. In Brody, T.M., Larner, J. and Minneman, K.P. (eds) *Human Pharmacology: Molecular to Clinical* (Third edition), (St. Louis: Mosby), 87–100.

Ehlert, F.J. (1998) Drugs affecting the parasympathetic nervous system and autonomic ganglia. In Brody, T.M., Larner, J. and Minneman, K.P. (eds) *Human Pharmacology: Molecular to Clinical* (Third edition), (St. Louis: Mosby), 101–118.

Martini, F.H. (1998) The autonomic nervous system. In Martini, F.H. *Fundamentals of Anatomy and Physiology* (Fourth edition), (New Jersey: Prentice Hall), 513–536.

Moore, K.E. (1998) Drugs affecting the sympathetic nervous system. In Brody, T.M., Larner, J. and Minneman, K.P. (eds) *Human Pharmacology: Molecular to Clinical* (Third edition), (St. Louis: Mosby), 119–141.

Rang, H.P., Dale, M.M. and Ritter, J.M. (1999) Chemical mediators and the autonomic nervous system. In Rang, H.P., Dale, M.M. and Ritter, J.M. *Pharmacology* (Fourth edition), (Edinburgh: Churchill Livingstone), 94–109.

Rang, H.P., Dale, M.M. and Ritter, J.M. (1999) Cholinergic transmission. In Rang, H.P., Dale, M.M. and Ritter, J.M. *Pharmacology* (Fourth edition), (Edinburgh: Churchill Livingstone), 110–138.

Rang, H.P., Dale, M.M. and Ritter, J.M. (1999) Local anaesthetics and drugs that effect ion channels. In Rang, H.P., Dale, M.M. and Ritter, J.M. *Pharmacology* (Fourth edition), (Edinburgh: Churchill Livingstone), 634–645.

Strichartz, G.R. (1998) Drugs affecting peripheral transmission: local anaesthetics. In Brody, T.M., Larner, J. and Minneman, K.P. (eds) *Human Pharmacology: Molecular to Clinical* (Third edition), (St. Louis: Mosby), 151–156.

■ COMPUTER-AIDED LEARNING PACKAGE

Further details of this learning package can be found at
http://www.coacs.com/PCCAL/

CardiovascularSystem/Autonomic Nervous System Tutor (version 3.0), Pharmacy Consortium for Computer Aided Learning (PCCAL), COACS Ltd, University of Bath.

THE CENTRAL NERVOUS SYSTEM AND DRUGS USED IN PSYCHIATRY

■ 3.1 INTRODUCTION

The brain and spinal cord can be thought of as an organ comprised of millions of individual nerve cells, each communicating with many other nerve cells. The mechanism of neurotransmission is discussed in Chapter 2. Each neuronal cell receives input from neighbouring cells, some of this input is inhibitory and some is excitatory. The response of the individual cell is therefore dependent upon the net effect of all of the incoming information. In general terms, drugs act on the central nervous system (CNS) to influence the balance of excitatory and inhibitory activity, thus drugs used to induce sleep or prevent 'over-activity' of the brain (for example convulsions) act by enhancing the actions of inhibitory neurotransmitters or decreasing the activity of excitatory neurotransmitters. Drugs used to treat conditions associated with 'under-activity' of the brain, for example depression, act by enhancing the activity of excitatory neurotransmitters or decreasing the actions of inhibitory neurotransmitters. The predominant inhibitory neurotransmitter in the brain is γ-aminobutyric acid (GABA); excitatory neurotransmitters include acetylcholine (ACh), 5-hydroxytryptamine (5-HT or serotonin) and noradrenaline (NA). In the UK, more prescription drugs are used for the treatment of psychiatric and other central nervous system disorders than are used for the treatment of conditions of any other system.

Drugs act on the central nervous system to influence the balance of activity of the excitatory and inhibitory neurotransmitters

■ 3.2 DRUGS THAT DECREASE CNS ACTIVITY

3.2.1 GENERAL ANAESTHETICS

General anaesthetics are drugs that cause a widespread decreased sensation and response to stimuli such as touch and pressure. Not all general anaesthetics reduce pain sensation and therefore they are sometimes used in combination with analgesics (see Section 3.2.2). The only therapeutic use of general anaesthetics is to permit surgery without the associated pain, discomfort and trauma. General anaesthetics are divided into two distict classes with different mechanisms of action and different uses. The two classes are the inhalation anaesthetics, which are either gases or vapours, and the intravenous anaesthetics.

3.2.1.1 Mechanism of action of general anaesthetics

There is still uncertainty about the precise mechanism of action of the inhalation general anaesthetics despite their therapeutic use since before 1850. It has long been recognised that the potency of general anaesthetics was directly related to their lipid solubility, thus

The potency of general anaesthetics is directly related to their lipid solubility, thus most lipid-soluble gases or vapours are able to induce anaesthesia

most lipid-soluble gases or vapours are able to induce anaesthesia. Of course, few such gases and vapours are used therapeutically because of other factors, such as toxicity and inflammability, but this has not prevented the 'street' use of agents such as solvents and cigarette-lighter fuel. The knowledge that the efficacy of an anaesthetic agent was related to its lipid solubility rather than its precise chemical structure led to the hypothesis that these drugs act by dissolving into, and disrupting the function of, the cell membrane. This 'lipid theory' proposes that the loss of function of the nerve cells occurs either because of an increase in the volume of the lipid component of the cells or an increase in the fluidity of the cell membrane. Such disruption of cell membrane properties is believed to result in the loss of function of some or all of the membrane-bound voltage- and ligand-gated ion channels (see Chapter 1). Experiments have demonstrated that these phenomena do, in fact, occur, but sometimes only at anaesthetic concentrations above those that are therapeutically effective; the relevance of these effects to therapeutic anaesthesia is therefore disputed.

An associated theory of inhalation anaesthetic action is the 'protein theory'. This theory proposes that the anaesthetics act by interacting directly with proteins within the cell membrane, most notably ion channels and receptor proteins. Experiments have shown that, at therapeutic concentrations, the anaesthetic agents are able to inhibit the actions of some receptors for excitatory transmitters and enhance the activity of some receptors for inhibitory transmitters. It is probable, however, that neither theory can fully explain the actions of all general anaesthetics, with some agents acting by dissolution into the lipid membrane, thereby disrupting membrane-bound protein function and some acting by direct interaction with the same membrane-bound proteins.

The mechanisms of action of the intravenous general anaesthetics, in contrast, is much more fully understood. The agents in question include benzodiazepines and barbiturates such as midazolam and thiopentone (thiopental), which act to enhance to effects of the inhibitory neurotransmitter GABA, and opioid receptor agonists such as fentanyl. The precise mechanisms of action of these drugs are described elsewhere in this chapter (see Sections 3.2.2, 3.2.3 and 3.2.4), but suffice it to say that they all act on well-recognised receptors, either to enhance or mimic the effects of inhibitory neurotransmitters or prevent the actions of excitatory transmitters.

3.2.1.2 The effects of general anaesthetics

Functions of the various brain areas are lost in a predictable order as the concentration of a CNS depressant agent, for example general anaesthetic, increases. The different degrees of loss of brain function induced by these agents have been labelled 'stages of anaesthesia'.

Stage I is called the stage of analgesia. In this stage the patient is still conscious but is drowsy and usually exhibits a reduced response to painful stimuli. Few medical procedures are performed during this stage of anaesthesia but it may be induced using nitrous oxide during childbirth. The benefit of this practice is that the patient remains conscious enough to self-administer the gas but gains sufficient pain relief. Halothane is of no such use because of its lack of analgesic effect.

Anaesthetics may cause loss of inhibition resulting in euphoria and uncontrolled laughing: 'laughing gas'

The second stage of anaesthesia is the stage of excitement. This stage occurs because inhibition is lost before consciousness. With nitrous oxide such loss of inhibition may result in euphoria and uncontrolled laughing, the reason behind the epithet 'laughing gas'; not all general anaesthetic agents possess such properties. As the patient passes further into the stage of excitement, consciousness is lost but reflexes become exaggerated, this may cause choking and vomiting and there may be incoherent talking and unpredictable, purposeless movement. This stage of anaesthesia is potentially dangerous not only to the patient but also to medical staff, thus anaesthetic practice aims to reduce its duration (see Section 3.2.1.4).

Stage III is surgical anaesthesia. At this stage reflexes are lost, respiration becomes regular and muscle tone is eventually lost. Loss of thoracic muscle tone eventually necessitates mechanical ventilation for the maintenence of breathing, and loss of vascular muscle tone may require administration of drugs to maintain blood pressure.

Stage IV represents medullary depression. At this stage respiratory and cardiovascular control is lost, usually resulting in death.

With the exception of stage IV, the patient again passes through each of the stages, but in reverse order, during recovery from anaesthesia.

3.2.1.3 Pharmacokinetics of general anaesthetic agents

The pharmacokinetics of inhalation anaesthetics are quite complicated, but an understanding of the factors that influence the absorption and distribution of these agents is important if the problems of induction and maintenance of anaesthesia are to be appreciated.

Unlike other drugs, the 'dose' of an inhalation anaesthetic is not expressed in terms of milligrams of drug, or even milligrams per kilogram of body weight, but in terms of partial pressure or percentage of inspired gas. The equivalent of ED_{50} for an inhalation anaesthetic is the Miminum Alveolar Concentration (MAC): the gaseous concentration of agent required to induce surgical anaesthesia in 50% of the population.

In a mixture of gases the partial pressure of each gas is proportional to the relative amounts, but where a gas is dissolved within a liquid (or tissue) the partial pressure is also dependent upon the solubility of the drug in that fluid. The partial pressure of a gas within a fluid is inversely proportional to the solubility of the drug in that fluid. If two drugs are present in a tissue at the same concentration, the drug with the higher solubility in that tissue will exert the lower partial pressure; it therefore follows that if two drugs are present in a tissue at the same partial pressure then the drug with the higher solubility will be present in a higher concentration. The degree of anaesthesia is dependent upon the concentration of anaesthetic in the brain.

All inhalation anaesthetics are highly lipid soluble and poorly water soluble. The driving force for the absorption and distribution of an inhalation anaesthetic is partial pressure, which, as discussed above, is dependent on the solubility of the drug in the fluid (tissue) concerned. Inhalation anaesthetics are administered via the lungs and the high partial pressure of the anaesthetic within the alveoli 'drives' the drug into the blood. Once in the blood the anaesthetics exert a relatively high partial pressure due to their poor aqueous solubility. This high pressure ensures that the gases are distributed to other compartments, most notably fats (lipids). At equilibrium the partial pressure of the anaesthetic in the alveoli, blood and lipids would be equal, but the concentration would be much greater in the lipid compartments.

The lipid compartment which receives the most anaesthetic is the brain, this is because the brain receives 75% of the cardiac output despite representing less than 10% of the body's mass. With time some of the anaesthetic redistributes to other lipid compartments (e.g. fat), but this can take several days as the fat receives only 5% of cardiac output despite representing nearly 20% of body mass. This knowledge is utilised when the concentration of anaesthetic gas or vapour administered is adjusted to take account of unusually high or low body weights. Cardiac output also needs to be considered: decreased cardiac output results in decreased perfusion of tissues such as muscle and fat, thereby increasing the concentration of anaesthetic agent that accumulates in the brain.

Because general anaesthesia is rarely maintained for a prolonged period of time, metabolism of the anaesthetic agent is of little therapeutic importance. Recovery from anaesthesia occurs because of redistribution of the drug away from the brain, usually back to the lungs for excretion. When the administration of the anaesthetic ceases, the partial pressure in the alveoli decreases; this results in diffusion of the drug from the blood to the alveoli, as a consequence of which more drug diffuses from the lipid compartment to the blood. In obese patients the time for recovery from anaesthesia may be increased because of the relatively greater distrubution of anaesthetic to fat stores, and therefore the relatively slower redistribution and excretion.

As the name implies, intravenous anaesthetics are administered directly into the bloodstream; the time taken to induce anaesthesia is therefore dependent solely on the time for the drug to move from the aqueous blood compartment to the lipid brain compartment. With drugs such as the barbiturate thiopentone (known as thiopental in USA) this may take just 20 seconds, whereas for benzodiazepines such as diazepam it would take several minutes. As described above, the rate of this distribution is governed by the lipid solubility. The high lipid solubility, however, also means that the drug is readily redistributed to other fat deposits, meaning that the duration of anaesthetic action of thiopentone is only 5–10 minutes. This drug is then slowly metabolised and excreted over the course of several hours. Repeated administration of thiopentone results in its accumulation in peripheral tissues, rendering maintenance of prolonged anaesthesia with thiopentone problematic. Two newer drugs, however, have advantages over thiopentone. Like thiopentone, etomidate and propofol are highly lipid soluble and are therefore rapid in their onset but short in duration of action, but these drugs are metabolised more rapidly than thiopentone. This means that etomidate and propofol have a lesser tendency to accumulate in peripheral tissues, to the extent that propofol can be used in the form of an infusion for maintained anaesthesia.

3.2.1.4 Anaesthetic practice

A list of commonly used inhalation and intravenous general anaesthetics is presented in Box 3.1. Following administration of an effective dose of an intravenous anaesthetic the patient passes through the stages of anaesthesia rapidly, but the duration of action of a single dose is short. For most intravenous anaesthetics maintenance of anaesthesia is not possible because of the problems described above, although it is possible to use infused propofol for relatively rapid, minor surgery. Inhalation anaesthetics allow maintenance of prolonged anaesthesia, which enables more major surgery, but they are slow in onset. This means that the patient remains conscious for several minutes while effective concentrations of the drug accumulate in the brain, and thus slowly passes through the stages of anaesthesia, notably the stage of excitement. Many patients find the process of using the face-mask traumatic and there is the risk of injury to both the patient and the medical staff during the stage of excitement. In order to overcome these problems it has become common to induce the anaesthesia with an intravenous agent, and then to maintain the anaesthesia with an inhalation agent. As presented in Box 3.1, several suitable inhalation anaesthetics are available but it is sometimes necessary to use a combination of two. A common combination is a mixture of halothane, nitrous oxide and oxygen. Nitrous oxide has good analgesic properties, but lacks the potency to induce unconsciousness, whereas halothane induces deep anaesthesia but has very poor analgesic properties. This combination induces the required depth of anaesthesia and provides good analgesia.

In addition to the anaesthetic agents themselves it is also common to administer other drugs either prior to the induction of the anaesthesia ('premedication') or along with

Patients may find the process of anaesthesia traumatic; it is therefore common to induce the anaesthesia rapidly with an intravenous agent, and then to maintain it with an inhalation agent

■ *Box 3.1* Properties of commonly available anaesthetic agents

Agent	Properties		Comments
	Potency	Speed of onset	
Inhalation anaesthetics			
Nitrous oxide	Low	Rapid	Good analgesic
Halothane	High	Moderate	No analgesia
Enflurane	Moderate	Moderate	
Isoflurane	Moderate	Moderate	Most commonly used
Intravenous anaesthetics			
Thiopentone (thiopental)		Fast	
Propofol	Greater than thiopentone	Fast	Can be used by infusion
Etomidate	As thiopentone	Fast	Safer than thiopentone
Ketamine		Moderate	
Midazolam		Slow	Benzodiazepine

the anaesthetic. Common premedications include benzodiazepines such as diazepam (see Section 3.2.4) which reduces the patient's anxiety, induces temporary amnesia, is a muscle relaxant and is itself anaesthetic in sufficient doses. All of these effects are beneficial in a patient about to undergo major surgery. Drugs such as antimuscarinic agents (Chapter 2) and histamine (H_2) antagonists (Chapter 7) may also be administered to prevent the secretion of saliva and gastric acid, which may interfere with the administration of the inhalation anaesthetic and may complicate the surgical procedure. Drugs such as analgesics (Section 3.2.2) may be given during the anaesthesia to provide extra pain relief, especially if the patient is also receiving neuromuscular blocking agents (Chapter 2) which are given to facilitate the surgery but also render the patient unable to respond to pain if the depth of anaesthesia is insufficient.

After anaesthesia the patient may receive additional analgesic cover, an anticholinesterase (Chapter 2) to reverse the effects of the neuromuscular blocking agent if one were used, and an antiemetic agent (Chapter 7) to relieve the nausea and vomiting induced by several anaesthetic agents (see Section 3.2.1.5).

3.2.1.5 Adverse effects of general anaesthetics

Many of the anaesthetics, both inhalation and intravenous, are associated with nausea and vomiting. There have also been reports of rare cases of liver damage and hyperthermia following halothane usage (due to release of sarcoplasmic calcium, causing prolonged muscle contraction), and teratogenic effects of nitrous oxide. The most serious danger of anaesthesia is overdosage, which invariably results in death. Another problem of inhalation anaesthetics relates not to the patient but to the medical staff. These agents are excreted by the patient unchanged, there is a risk therefore of the operating theatre atmosphere becoming contaminated with anaesthetic agent. This not only renders the staff susceptible to the sedative effects but also to the longer-term effects such as liver toxicity and damage to an unborn fetus.

There is a risk of the operating theatre atmosphere becoming contaminated with anaesthetic agent, rendering the staff susceptible to the sedative effects

■ *Box 3.2* Opioid agents and their properties

Agent	*Properties*
Morphine	The most valuable opioid analgesic. Morphine also induces euphoria, respiratory depression, constipation, etc.
Diamorphine (heroin)	Highly potent analgesic; more highly soluble than morphine, allowing administration of higher doses in smaller volumes
Codeine	Effective against mild to moderate pain. Useful as antidiarrhoeal agent and cough suppressant
Methadone	Less sedating than morphine, with longer duration of action. Used to assist withdrawal from morphine or heroin
Pethidine	Short-acting analgesic, less potent than morphine
Fentanyl	Rapid onset, short-acting analgesic used in general anaesthesia

■ 3.2.2 NARCOTIC ANALGESICS

As described in Section 3.2.1, the term anaesthetic refers to a compound which removes sensations such as touch and pressure, some anaesthetics also inhibit the pain sensation. Drugs which are able to inhibit the pain sensation without affecting the other sensory modalities are known as analgesics. There are two pharmacologically distinct classes of analgesic drugs: the non-steroidal anti-inflammatory drugs (see Chapter 9) and the narcotic analgesics. Narcotic analgesics are drugs which are related in their mechanism of action to morphine; such drugs are more correctly termed opioid analgesics, to indicate their similarities to the extracts of the opium poppy: morphine and codeine. Some of the members of the opioid family are presented in Box 3.2.

Analgesics are drugs that are able to inhibit the pain sensation without affecting the other sensory modalities

All of the opioid agents act on the same group of seven transmembrane domain, G-protein coupled receptors. Activation of the opioid receptors results in a decrease in the synthesis of cAMP, via G_i, opening of potassium channels or closing of calcium channels; all of these effects are therefore inhibitory. Opioid receptors can be divided into three major subgroups: μ (mu), δ (delta) and κ (kappa) receptors. The most important of these receptors are the μ receptors, which are found in those areas of the brain concerned with pain perception (periaqueductal grey matter, locus ceruleus and thalamus), in the spinal cord and in the gut. Activation of the μ receptors reduces the release of other transmitters involved in pain sensation and leads to analgesia, euphoria, sedation, respiratory depression, suppression of the cough reflex, nausea and vomiting.

κ receptors are located in the thalamus and the dorsal horn of spinal cord. These receptors also produce analgesia, but in a manner independent of the effects of the μ receptors. Unlike the μ receptors, κ receptors produce dysphoric rather than euphoric effects. δ receptors are also found in the brain and spinal cord and are concerned with analgesia.

One of the most exciting pharmacological discoveries of the latter half of the twentieth century was the identification of the endogenous agonists for the opioid receptors. Three groups of endogenous opioid agonists were found, these were the endorphins, the enkephalins and the dynorphins; the names were derived the term 'endogenous morphine' and the Greek for 'in the head' and 'powerful', respectively. Endorphins are long peptides; β-endorphin, for example, is a 31-amino-acid chain which is derived from the same precursor as adrenocorticotrophic hormone (ACTH) and melanocyte stimulating

• **Figure 3.1** A comparison of the amino acid sequences of the endorphins, enkephalins and related substances

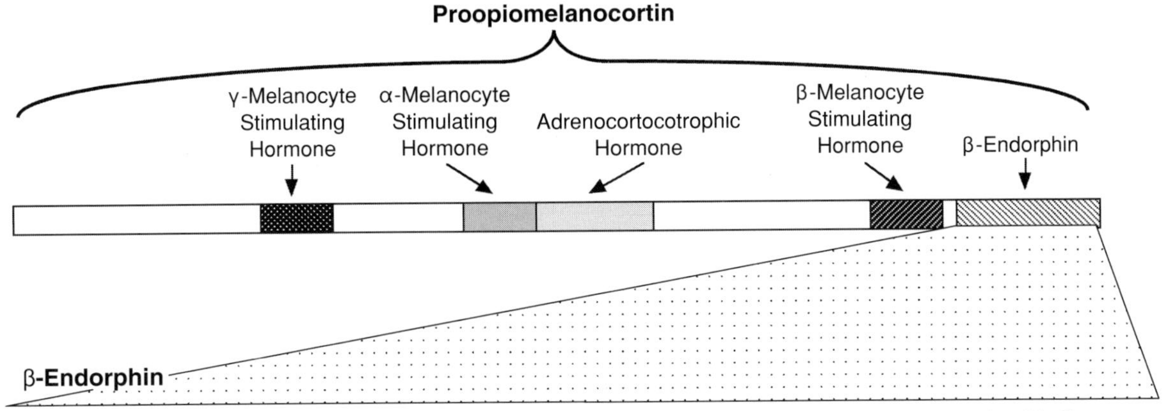

Proopiomelanocortin

γ-Melanocyte Stimulating Hormone

α-Melanocyte Stimulating Hormone

Adrenocortocotrophic Hormone

β-Melanocyte Stimulating Hormone

β-Endorphin

β-Endorphin

Tyr-Gly-Gly-Phe-Met-Thr-Ser-Glu-Lys-Ser-Gln-Thr-Pro--Leu-Val-Thr-Leu-Phe-Lys-Asn-Ala-Ile-Ile-Lys-Asn-Ala-Tyr-Lys-Lys-Gly-Glu

Dynorphin
Tyr-Gly-Gly-Phe-Leu-Arg-Aeg-Ile-Arg-Pro-Lys-Leu-Lys-Trp-Asp-Asn-Gln

Met-enkephalin
Tyr-Gly-Gly-Phe-Met

Leu-enkephalin
Tyr-Gly-Gly-Phe-Leu

hormone (MSH). β-Endorphin contains within its structure the same amino acid sequence as methionine-enkephalin (see figure 3.1). β-Endorphin is found in the hypothalamus and the anterior pituitary gland, and is released at times of stress. The principal enkephalins are leucine-enkephalin and methionine-enkephalin, two pentapeptides which are found throughout the CNS and gastrointestinal tract (see figure 3.1). The final endogenous opioid agonists are the dynorphins, these are again found within the CNS, most notably the hypothalamus and posterior pituitary gland. Dynorphin A contains within its structure the amino acid sequence of leucine-enkephalin.

The normal physiological role of the endogenous opioid agonists is the inhibition of pain (figure 3.2). Pain is detected in the periphery by specialised nociceptors, the action potential generated by these receptors is then carried to the dorsal horn of the spinal cord in either small, myelinated Aδ fibres or in larger, more slowly conducting C fibres. Within the spinal cord these action potentials cause the release of excitatory neuro-transmitters, such as substance P, which generate further action potentials within the spinothalamic tract, which then carries the nerve impulses to the brain. To modulate the afferent pain impulses, however, action potentials are generated within the periaqueductal grey matter of the midbrain. These impulses are carried down the spinal cord to the dorsal horn where they cause the release of neurotransmitters which act to inhibit the transmission of the primary pain impulse from the Aδ fibres and C fibres to the spinothalamic tract. Amongst the inhibitory neurotransmitters utilised within the periaqueductal grey matter and the dorsal horn of the spinal cord are the endogenous opioid agonists.

The opioids that are used therapeutically all act by mimicking the endogenous pain-modulating peptides. The differences between the various opioid analgesics are related primarily to their pharmacokinetics, but also to their relative actions on the different

The normal physiological role of the endogenous opioids is the inhibition of pain

41

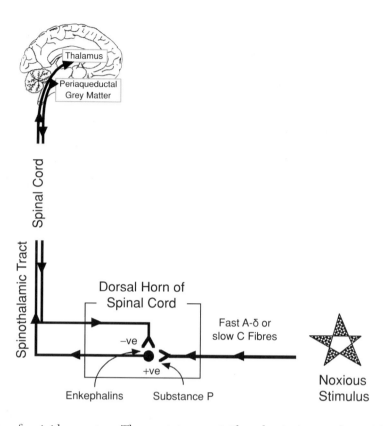

• **Figure 3.2** A representation of the primary nervous pathways involved with the perception of pain

subtypes of opioid receptor. The prototype opioid analgesic is morphine. Morphine acts on μ receptors to induce effective analgesia, this analgesia may be used to prevent the pain during and after surgery, or it may be used to prevent pain in terminal illness (for example cancer). In addition to the pain relief, morphine may also cause sedation and euphoria. Morphine also acts in the medulla oblongata to supress the cough reflex and acts in the gut to inhibit gut motility, it may therefore be used to relieve cough and diarrhoea.

Morphine inhibits pain, causes euphoria, suppresses cough and inhibits gut motility

In clinical usage the different morphine-like agents are selected according to the properties required. Fentanyl and pethidine, for example, produce rapid-onset, but short-acting, analgesia. They are therefore used for analgesia and anaesthesia related to surgery and childbirth. Diamorphine (heroin) is metabolised to morphine and produces equivalent analgesia; it has advantages over morphine in that it induces a lesser degree of nausea and has greater water solubility, which facilitates administration. Codeine produces much less analgesia than morphine, and therefore can only be used for the treatment of mild pain; it does, however, effectively suppress the cough reflex and therefore may be used therapeutically for that purpose. Loperamide crosses the blood–brain barrier very slowly and is therefore of little use as a cough suppressant or analgesic; it does, however, have profound effects on the gut, rendering it useful for the relief of diarrhoea. Methadone has a much greater duration of action than morphine, it therefore does not cause the sudden euphoria on administration followed by the dysphoria as the effects subside. Methadone is used in the treatment of opioid addiction, partly because it prevents the euphoric effects of morphine if the two drugs are used simultaneously, a direct consequence of the two drugs acting via the same receptors, and partly because its longer plasma half-life reduces the problems of withdrawal effects.

Despite their exceptional clinical usefulness, there are also many problems associated with the opioid analgesics. The most important adverse effect of opioids is respiratory depression. Opioids reduce the sensitivity of the brainstem to carbon dioxide, and therefore remove the stimulus to breathe. All of the opioid analgesics that cross the blood–brain barrier have the potential to suppress respiration, and thus respiratory depression is the major cause of death following overdose. The other adverse properties of opioids are related to their tendency to cause tolerance and dependence. Tolerance refers to the phenomenon where increasing doses of the drug are required to produce the same effect. The cellular mechanism of opioid tolerance is not understood, but the consequence of tolerance is that an initial starting dose of morphine of 40mg/day may need to rise gradually to 1g/day with continued use. Dependence is the phenomenon in which the body adapts to the continued presence of the drug; removal of the drug therefore precipitates a state of 'abnormality' characterised by withdrawal or abstinence symptoms. In the case of opioids, the withdrawal effects include increased sensitivity to pain, cough, diarrhoea and depression. These unpleasant withdrawal symptoms are alleviated by further administration of an opioid: the basis of addiction. It should be remembered that because the opioid analgesics all act via the same receptors there is cross-tolerance, and that the withdrawal effects precipitated by abstinence from one opioid can be relieved by administration of another.

Overdose with an opioid can be treated by administration of a competitive antagonist of opioid receptors, such as naloxone, these agents reverse the effects of the opioid agonists but therefore also precipitate the onset of the withdrawal effects.

■ 3.2.3 ANTICONVULSANT AGENTS

Convulsions or seizures are characterised by occasional, high frequency electrical discharges of groups of neurones in the brain. The symptoms experienced by the patient depend on which neurones are affected, thus firing of neurones of the cerebral cortex may cause uncontrolled motor activity or abnormal sensory experiences, whereas firing of neurones of the brainstem may cause loss of consciousness. Epilepsy is defined as the presence of recurrent, self-limiting seizures.

There are two main categories of epileptic seizures: partial and generalised. Partial seizures are those discharges of electrical activity which affect distinct groups of neurones and which remain localised. The symptoms of such seizures may involve repetitive contractions of a single group of muscles, or abnormal sensations such as hearing voices or seeing coloured lights. Some partial seizures result in quite complex arrays of abnormal behaviour, such as purposeless hand-rubbing. Generalised seizures occur when the abnormal electrical activity involves the whole brain, the characteristic feature here is a loss of consciousness. Generalised seizures may result in repeated muscle contractions throughout the whole body (grand mal epilepsy) or may simply involve sudden, short-lived loss of consciousness (petit mal epilepsy). The aim of the treatment for epilepsy is to prevent the occurrence of seizures without inducing undue adverse effects such as sedation.

All anticonvulsant drugs act by decreasing neuronal activity; this is achieved either by stabilising the neuronal membrane, thus preventing rapidly repeating depolarisations, or by enhancing the actions of inhibitory neurotransmitters such as GABA. One of the earliest drugs used in the treatment of epilepsy was phenobarbitone (phenobarbital). Barbiturates such as phenobarbitone act via a receptor linked to the $GABA_A$ receptor–chloride ion channel complex (figure 3.3). GABA normally acts on its receptor to induce the opening of a chloride ion channel; the resultant movement of chloride ions into the

• **Figure 3.3** A representation of a chloride ion channel and associated receptors. GABA acts to open the ion channel, benzodiazepines and barbiturates act to potentiate the effects of GABA

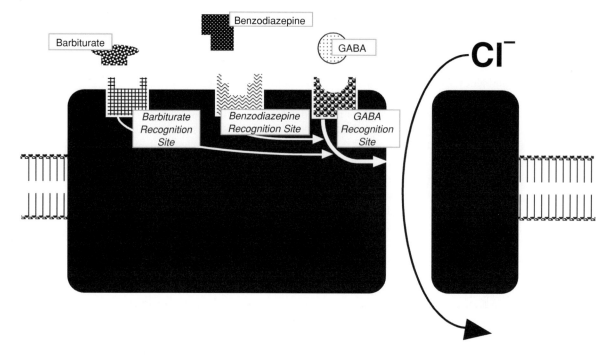

cell along the concentration gradient increases the membrane potential and therefore makes depolarisation of the membrane less likely. Barbiturates bind to a receptor which is separate from the GABA receptor, but the stimulation of which potentiates the effect of GABA on the movement of chloride ions. Phenobarbitone, and the related compound primidone, are capable of reducing the duration and intensity of generalised seizures but have no beneficial effect against absence seizures. The clinical usefulness of these compounds, however, is limited by their sedative effects.

The benzodiazepine drugs diazepam, clonazepam and clobazam act in a manner similar to the barbiturates. They bind to a specific benzodiazepine receptor which is associated with the $GABA_A$ receptor–chloride ion channel complex; like barbiturates the benzodiazepines potentiate the effects of GABA. Benzodiazepines may be used in the treatment of epilepsy, but like barbiturates their effectiveness is limited by their sedative effects. One exception to this is the treatment of status epilepticus, a condition in which several seizures occur consecutively without consciousness being regained, benzodiazepines are the treatment of choice for status epilepticus.

Drugs such as carbamazepine selectively block repetitively active ion channels, thus they permit the initial action potential but prevent high-frequency firing

The other mechanism of action of anticonvulsant agents is the stabilisation of the neuronal membrane. Drugs such as carbamazepine, phenytoin and lamotrigine prevent the opening of voltage-gated sodium ion channels, and therefore prevent the development and propagation of action potentials. The important feature of these compounds is that they act selectively on repetitively active ion channels, thus they permit the initial action potential but prevent high-frequency firing. Carbamazepine and phenytoin are effective only against grand mal seizure, but valproate is also effective against petit mal seizure, possibly because of an action on a particular subtype of sodium channels.

Another drug useful in the treatment of petit mal epilepsy is ethosuximide, this agent is ineffective against tonic–clonic (repetitive muscle contraction and relaxation) seizures.

■ *Box 3.3* Commonly used anticonvulsant agents

Mechanism of action	Agent	Proprietary name
Agents acting at the GABA receptor	Phenobarbitone (phenobarbital)	Phenobarbitone (phenobarbital)
	Primidone	Mysoline®
	Clonazepam	Rivotril®
	Clobazam	Frisium®
	Diazepam	Diazemuls®
Neuronal membrane stabilizers	Carbamazepine	Tegretol®
	Sodium valproate	Epilim®
	Phenytoin	Epanutin®
Other	Vigabatrin	Sabril®
	Tiagabine	Gabitril®

The mechanism of action of ethosuximide may be dependent upon inhibition of a particular subtype of calcium channel.

Sodium valproate is effective against most forms of seizure. This drug acts by increasing the effects of GABA, possibly by preventing its metabolism, although it also has effects on sodium ion channels similar to those of phenytoin. More recent advances in the treatment of epilepsy have been the development of agents such as vigabatrin, which also increases GABA activity by inhibiting the enzyme responsible for the breakdown of GABA, and tiagabine which prevents reuptake of GABA into the presynaptic terminal. Examples of some common anticonvulsant agents are presented in Box 3.3.

■ **3.2.4 DRUGS USED IN THE TREATMENT OF ANXIETY**

Anxiety is a normal aspect of human mood, it is usually accompanied by autonomic changes such as increased heart rate, sweating and relaxation of the gastrointestinal tract. Severe stress or anxiety induces increased muscle tone, irritability and, if continued, fatigue. These symptoms, however, become a clinical problem if they are prolonged and/or if they prevent individuals from carrying out their normal duties and functions. In many cases individuals who are anxious self-medicate using sedative agents such as alcohol, these agents mask the anxiety but at the expense of sedation and possibly even motor incoordination.

Anxiolytic drugs are agents which are able to alleviate the anxiety without inducing sedation. The most widely used anxiolytic drugs are the benzodiazepines, such as diazepam and chlordiazepoxide (see Box 3.4). As described in Section 3.2.3, benzodiazepines act by potentiating the effects of the inhibitory neurotransmitter GABA, they therefore potentiate inhibition within the brain. There is little difference in the effects of the different benzodiazepines, other than differences in pharmacokinetics. Diazepam, for example, has a duration of action of 24–48 hours while lorazepam has only 18 hours' activity. The choice of agent is dependent on the condition being treated, whether the drug is being used for prevention of the short-term anxiety associated with a surgical procedure or an examination, or whether it is being used for the relief of a chronic condition. In terms of adverse effects, the benzodiazepines are relatively free of adverse effects, the most troublesome being sedation. The sedative effect of these drugs is a function of dose, and therefore undue sedation can be reduced by a decrease in dose. In cases of

■ *Box 3.4* The properties and actions of anxiolytic agents

Classification	Agent	Proprietary name
Sustained action benzodiazepines	Diazepam	Valium®
	Chlordiazepoxide	Librium®
	Alprazolam	Xanax®
Short-acting benzodiazepines	Lorazepam	Ativan®
5-HT$_{1A}$ receptor agonist	Buspirone	Buspar®

overdose, the sedation can be reversed using the benzodiazepine receptor antagonist, flumazenil. A major concern about the use of these drugs arises from their tendency to induce tolerance and dependence. With continued use these drugs require increasing doses to elicit the same response; on cessation of treatment the patient may then suffer rebound anxiety and insomnia. Withdrawal from benzodiazepines also occasionally induces bizarre perceptual (visual) distortions. These withdrawal effects often precipitate continued use of the agents for many years. It is now recognised that benzodiazepines should only be used for the short-term relief of anxiety, but even a single dose of short-acting, i.e. rapid off-set, benzodiazepines has been associated with rebound effects.

Another drug used for the relief of anxiety is buspirone. Buspirone is an agonist at 5-HT$_{1A}$ receptors, although whether this is the mechanism by which it relieves anxiety is unclear as the clinical effects are not seen for several days after initiation of treatment. Buspirone does not cause sedation and it does not relieve the symptoms associated with withdrawal from benzodiazepines; the two types of anxiolytics therefore appear to have independent mechanisms of action. There is, as yet, insufficient evidence to allow the liability of buspirone to cause dependence to be assessed.

Other drugs that have been used to relieve anxiety include the β-adrenoceptor antagonist propranolol and barbiturates. Propranolol acts by reducing the autonomic manifestations of anxiety, for example tachycardia, the individual therefore feels calmer. Propranolol is not acting centrally in the relief of anxiety. Barbiturates relieve anxiety by virtue of their sedative effects, which, as described in Section 3.2.3, like those of benzodiazepines are mediated by potentiation of the effects of GABA at the chloride ion channel. Barbiturates are no longer used for the relief of anxiety because of their lethal effects in overdose and their liability to induce tolerance and dependence.

■ 3.2.5 DRUGS USED TO INDUCE SLEEP

Insomnia is rarely a disorder in its own right, it is normally a symptom of some other condition: difficulty in getting to sleep, for example, may be caused by excessive anxiety, whereas early morning wakening may be a symptom of depression. The drugs used in the relief of insomnia, termed hypnotics, are generally short to medium acting, so that they enable the person to fall asleep, but their action is not so long as to present problems of awakening at the appropriate time. The most common drugs used for the treatment of insomnia are benzodiazepines; as described in Section 3.2.3, these agents act on specific receptors to enhance the actions of the inhibitory neurotransmitter GABA on the chloride ion channel. Two newer drugs, zolpidem and zopiclone, are chemically unrelated to the benzodiazepines but act via the same receptors. Other drugs used as hypnotics are anticholinergic agents such as diphenhydramine (which is an antihistamine with antimuscarinic actions) and ethanol, which depresses neuronal activity either by

■ *Box 3.5* Commonly used hypnotic agents and their properties

Agent	*Proprietary name*
Nitrazepam	Mogadon®
Flunitrazepam	Rohypnol®
Flurazepam	Dalmane®
Zolpidem	Stilnoct®
Zopiclone	Zimovane®

disruption of cell membrane activity or by direct actions on membrane-bound ion channels. The two latter agents are used either as self-medication (diphenhydramine, for example, is available 'over-the-counter' as Nytol®), or as an 'informal' medication, as is the case for ethanol which is often administered to elderly patients in nursing homes in the form of a 'night-cap'.

All hypnotics depress CNS activity; this might be seen as an appropriate property for such drugs, but it should be remembered that the brain is not inactive during sleep. Approximately 20–25% of normal sleep is stage V sleep, also called 'rapid eye movement' or REM sleep. During REM sleep the brain is paradoxically active and the eyes move rapidly beneath the closed eyelids. If the subject is awakened from REM sleep, he or she reports dreaming. REM sleep is believed to be the most 'refreshing' component of sleep. The duration and frequency of REM sleep increases later in the sleep period, thus typically it is greatest just before wakening. If subjects are deprived of REM sleep, but allowed the other sleep stages, they awake unrefreshed, and, if the deprivation is prolonged, may start to exhibit psychological disorders. The proportion of REM sleep is increased in sleep which follows a period of REM deprivation, thus there appears to be some form of 'catch-up' phenomenon. As outlined above, REM sleep is associated with dreaming and subjects report abnormally vivid dreams or nightmares during the sleep that follows periods of REM deprivation.

Because of their CNS depressant effects, hypnotic agents have a tendency to depress REM sleep. The ideal hypnotic agent, therefore, is one which acts for long enough to allow the individual to get to sleep, but does not act long enough to depress REM sleep. The properties of various hypnotic agents are presented in Box 3.5. It is generally considered that hypnotic agents should not be used for long periods of time, with the maximum being about 2 weeks. An alternative approach is to use the agents intermittently, as required, so that REM deprivation and subsequent rebound increased REM does not occur.

Cessation of hypnotic therapy may be associated with increased vividness of dreams due to a rebound increase in REM sleep

■ 3.2.6 DRUGS USED TO TREAT MANIA

Mania is a condition in which an individual is abnormally elated, enthusiastic and optimistic, it may last for several days or several months. The affected person is typically excessively loud and rapid in speech, and may make inappropriate demands upon friends' time. During the episode of mania the person may also make, and put into action, grandiose and obviously unrealist plans, such as investing large amounts of money in unwise business ventures. Another common symptom is excessive spending, for example ordering a brand new luxury motor car, in the absence of adequate financial resources. The mania, however, is not always 'good-willed', so that it may be characterised by excessive irritability and outbursts of anger.

In some patients the episodes of mania alternate with periods of depression (see Section 3.3.1); this condition is known as manic depression or bipolar disorder and is characterised by swings of mood from mania to depression which in some cases may occur very suddenly and/or may occur frequently, for example at weekly or monthly intervals.

Acute episodes of mania may be treated with benzodiazepines (see Sections 3.2.3, 3.2.4, 3.2.5), carbamazepine (see Section 3.2.3) or antipsychotic agents (see Section 3.2.7), but the most commonly used drug for the treatment and prevention of mania is lithium (for example Priadel®, Liskonum®). Lithium is also effective in the relief of bipolar disorder where it appears to 'stabilise' mood. The mechanism of this monovalent cation is unknown, although lithium can pass through voltage-gated sodium ion channels but is not a substrate for the sodium–potassium ATPase pump. The most probable mechanism of action of lithium in the treatment of mania relates to its inhibitory effects on the synthesis of the intracellular second messengers cAMP and inositol triphosphate (IP_3).

> Lithium stabilises mood in manic depression and is also effective in the treatment of both mania and depression when they occur independently

The major problem with the use of lithium is its toxicity. Lithium has a very narrow therapeutic window and in overdose may cause tremor, confusion, convulsions or death. In lower concentrations lithium induces excessive thirst (polydipsia) due to effects on the kidney related to sodium retention and inhibition of the actions of antidiuretic hormone, and may cause thyroid gland dysfunction.

■ 3.2.7 DRUGS USED IN THE TREATMENT OF PSYCHOSES

The term psychosis refers to an extreme degree of behavioural and/or cognitive disorder. Conditions such as anxiety, mania and depression (see Sections 3.2.4, 3.2.6 and 3.3.1, respectively) are disorders of mood in which the individual retains a 'sense of reality', that means that the person usually recognises that they are ill and that their feelings are not normal. Such conditions are termed 'affective disorders'. In pychoses the individual may exhibit symptoms of profound anxiety, depression or mania, but 'loses touch with reality'. The archetypal form of pyschosis is schizophrenia, although there are other psychotic illnesses.

The symptoms of schizophrenia are usually divided into 'positive' symptoms and 'negative' symptoms. Positive symptoms are symptoms such as hallucinations, which are usually auditory, and delusions, for example delusions of grandeur or paranoid delusions. The negative symptoms are features such as social withdrawal and lack of purposeful behaviour. There may also be cognitive disruption so that speech and written communication is comprised of 'word salads': strings of words with no rational meaning. Many schizophrenic individuals ascribe their thought patterns to religious experiences (hearing the word of God) or particular artistic sensitivity (being able to appreciate the hidden meaning of poems, novels, pictures, etc.). Positive and negative symptoms usually occur together, thus these individuals are socially withdrawn and have difficulty maintaining relationships, and may have the belief that they are being constantly followed and monitored by one of their neighbours. There are, historically, several cases where individuals have committed crimes such as murder or abduction, but in their defence have stated that they were acting on the instruction of 'voices in their head'. Usually, if the personal history of such people is studied it is apparent that they are not fully integrated into society, have difficulty with personal relationships, and have previously exhibited bizarre behaviour or have expressed bizarre ideas in speech, text or art. Approximately 1% of the population is diagnosed as schizophrenic, usually before the age of 25.

> It is not clear what causes schizophrenia, but most of the drugs that are effective in its treatment are antagonists of the dopamine receptor

It is not clear what causes schizophrenia, but most of the drugs that are effective in its treatment are antagonists of the dopamine (D_2) receptor. Most antipsychotic agents, however, also possess antagonistic properties at muscarinic receptors, adrenoceptors,

■ *Box 3.6* Antipsychotic agents and their properties

Agent	Proprietary name	Properties
Chlorpromazine	Largactil®	Highly sedating
Droperidol	Droleptan®	
Flupenthixol (flupentixol)	Depixol®	Depot injection for 2-weekly dosing; less sedating than chlorpromazine
Haloperidol	Serenace®	Greater incidence of extrapyramidal symptoms than chlorpromazine
Loxapine	Loxapac®	Low tendency to cause sedation
Clozapine	Clozaril®	Used in patients who are unresponsive to other treatments
Risperidone	Risperdal®	Effective against both positive and negative symptoms

serotonin receptors and histamine receptors. It is the fact that there is a very good linear correlation between the therapeutic efficacy of an antipsychotic agent and its ability to antagonise the D_2 receptor that sustains the 'dopamine hypothesis' of schizophrenia. This hypothesis states that the illness is caused by an overactivity of the dopaminergic neurones of the midbrain and that it is treated by dopamine antagonism. Newer drugs used for the treatment of schizophrenia, for example clozapine and resperidone, have reduced affinity for the D_2 receptor, but have high affinity for the $5\text{-}HT_2$ receptor, thus questioning the dopamine hypothesis; clozapine is also an antagonist at the D_4 receptor.

Drugs used for the treatment of psychoses are presented in Box 3.6. Approximately 70% of schizophrenic patients experience a lessening of the symptoms when they use these drugs, but the effects are greater against the positive than the negative symptoms. Risperidone is seen to be effective against both positive and negative symptoms. All antipsychotic agents have a sedating effect, but one which is qualitatively different from the sedation induced by benzodiazepines and barbiturates. Antipsychotic agents rapidly induce a state in which the patient fails to respond to the environment or to show emotion, but when roused they are able to respond to questions accurately. Although this sedating effect is rapid in onset, the relief of the schizophrenia takes several weeks; this suggests that the two effects are not mediated by the same mechanism of action. In many respects it is the efficacy of the antipsychotic agents in the treatment of the symptoms that results in the high incidence of relapse. Patients improve while using the medication, they therefore regain rational thought. One consequence of this is that the patients believe themself to be cured and therefore no longer in need of medication. This rationalised non-compliance to the medication results in the psychiatric relapse. To overcome this problem some antipsychotic agents are administered in the form of depot injections that are given every 2–4 weeks, for example flupenthixol (Depixol®).

The major concern with the antipsychotic agents is their tendency to cause adverse effects. The antagonism of muscarinic receptors may contribute to the sedative actions but also induces the classic symptoms of dry mouth, blurred vision, urinary retention, constipation and tachycardia. The antagonism of α-adrenoceptors is responsible for hypotension and postural hypotension, while antagonism of 5-HT receptors may explain the induced hypothermia. Antagonism of the dopamine receptors is responsible for the most serious adverse effects. Dopamine antagonism causes secretion of prolactin, resulting in reduced fertility, menstrual disorders and possible gynaecomastia and galactorrhoea (breast development in males and abnormal milk production). Dopamine antagonism also disrupts the extrapyramidal system of the brain. This brain area is responsible for the control of fine motor control, thus the extrapyramidal side-effects are characterised by abnormal voluntary movement with tremor and restlessness. These symptoms are analogous to those seen in Parkinson's disease (see Section 3.3.2). A second extrapyramidal side-effect is tardive dyskinesia, a condition in which there are repetitive abnormal movements of the face and tongue (chewing and licking-like movements). The Parkinson's-like symptoms are a direct consequence of dopamine receptor antagonism and usually onset within the first few weeks of antipsychotic drug therapy. These symptoms may be reduced by a lowering of the dose of antipsychotic agent used or by co-administration of a muscarinic antagonist. Ironically, those antipsychotic agents with pronounced effects on muscarinic receptors are therefore less likely to induce extrapyramidal side-effects than those agents with greater selectivity for the D_2 receptor. The tardive dyskinesia is slower in onset, is irreversible and does not respond to antimuscarinic drugs; its cause is unclear but may be related to the expression of novel D_2 receptors as a consequence of chronic receptor antagonism.

■ 3.3 DRUGS THAT INCREASE CNS ACTIVITY
3.3.1 ANTIDEPRESSANT AGENTS

Depressive illness is the most common psychiatric illness, affecting approximately 10% of the population at some point in their lives. Depression or sadness is a normal response to everyday events, and is therefore a normal emotion. Typical symptoms of depression are feelings of pessimism with decreased self-esteem. There may also be feelings of guilt, although the subject does not know of what they are guilty! The physical signs of depression are loss of appetite and libido with insomnia, coupled with early morning wakening. There may also be autonomic symptoms such as constipation and decreased body temperature. The differentiation between the normal emotion of sadness and depressive illness depends on the severity of the symptoms, their duration and the presence or absence of any triggering event. For example depression is not unexpected following bereavement, but would be considered abnormal if it were still present 1 year later. Depression following an identifiable trigger event, sometimes called a life event, is called reactive depression and is often considered to be better treated with counselling than with drugs. Depression with no identifiable trigger is called endogenous depression, and is usually treated with antidepressant drugs.

The biochemical cause of endogenous depression is unknown, although the most prominent theory is the 'monoamine theory of depression'. This theory states that depression is caused by a deficiency of one or both of the monoamines serotonin and noradrenaline. Antidepressant drugs act by increasing the functional concentrations of these neurotransmitters. There is a great deal of evidence both for and against this theory, but suffice to say that it still serves as a good basis for the understanding of the mechanism of action of antidepressant drugs.

The first antidepressant drugs were developed following the observation that the antitubercular drug isoniazid elevated mood in depressed patients, this led to the introduction of the isoniazid analogue iproniazid for the treatment of depression. It was subsequently shown that isoniazid and iproniazid inhibit the actions of the enzyme monoamine oxidase. This enzyme is normally responsible, amongst other things, for the metabolism and inactivation of both noradrenaline and serotonin in the CNS. It therefore follows

■ *Box 3.7* The properties and actions of commonly used antidepressant drugs

Classification	Agent	Proprietary name
Monoamine oxidase inhibitor (MAOI)	Phenelzine	Nardil®
	Tranylcypromine	Parnate®
Reversible MAOI	Moclobemide	Manerix®
Tricyclic antidepressant	Amitriptyline	Lentizol®
	Imipramine	Tofranil®
	Doxepin	Sinequan®
Selective serotonin re-uptake inhibitors	Fluoxetine	Prozac®
	Fluvoxamine	Faverin®
Selective noradrenaline re-uptake inhibitors	Reboxetine	Edronax®

that inhibition of monoamine oxidase leads to an increase in serotonergic and noradrenergic function in the CNS. Non-competitive, irreversible monoamine oxidase inhibitors (MAOIs) are now widely available for the treatment of depression (see Box 3.7), and a recent advance has been the introduction of moclobemide, a reversible inhibitor of monoamine oxidase subtype A (RIMA). This drug inhibits the enzyme subtype that is responsible for the breakdown of serotonin and noradrenaline, but has no effect on MAO B, which is reponsible for the breakdown of dopamine. This selectivity of action reduces the side-effects.

MAOIs cause adverse effects predominantly because of the inhibition of such a ubiquitous enzyme. Monoamine oxidase is a normal hepatic enzyme involved in the metabolism of dietary amines. If the enzyme is inhibited then some of these amines, most notably tyramine, are absorbed unchanged. Tyramine is an indirectly acting sympathomimetic, thus it causes the release of noradrenaline. This action itself would induce side-effects, but because of the presence of the MAOI the action of the released noradrenaline is enhanced. The overt effect of these events is a dangerous rise in blood pressure accompanied by a severe headache. Because cheese contains large amounts of tyramine, this is often referred to as the 'cheese effect', and patients receiving MAOIs are warned not to eat cheese. Other foodstuffs that contain tyramine, and therefore pose the same risks, are broad beans, yeast extracts, meat extracts and soya extracts.

Patients receiving monoamine oxidase inhibitors are warned not to eat cheese, broad beans, Marmite or caviar

Other side-effects of MAOIs relate to their anticholinergic actions, thus they have a tendency to cause sedation, dry mouth, constipation, etc. MAOIs may also cause insomnia, presumably because of the effects on the CNS of serotonin and noradrenaline; whether the sedation or the insomnia predominates appears to depend on the age of the patient (sedation is greatest in the elderly) and the time of day that the drug is administered.

The most commonly used antidepressant drugs are the tricyclic antidepressants, so called because of their generic chemical structure. These drugs have been shown to inhibit the re-uptake of noradrenaline and serotonin into the presynaptic nerve terminal. Neuronal re-uptake is more important than MAO in the inactivation of these neurotransmitters. Since the initial introduction of the tricyclic antidepressant drugs, several other compounds have been developed with the same actions, but which are not chemically related. A better name for this class of drug is therefore 're-uptake inhibitors' (see Box 3.7). Re-uptake inhibitors vary in their ability to inhibit the re-uptake of serotonin and noradrenaline, thus some are equi-effective in preventing re-uptake of both

Prozac® is a selective
serotonin re-uptake
inhibitor

neurotransmitters, whereas others prevent only serotonin reuptake: the so-called selective serotonin re-uptake inhibitors (SSRIs). Reboxetine (Edronax®) inhibits only noradrenaline reuptake. There is little evidence to suggest that these drugs differ greatly in their ability to relieve depression, but they do differ in the profiles of their adverse effects.

Those antidepressant drugs that prevent noradrenaline re-uptake in the CNS may also prevent noradrenaline re-uptake in the heart. Such drugs have a tendency to cause arrythmias and heart block. SSRIs have little or no tendency to produce adverse cardiac effects. Many antidepressant drugs also possess anticholinergic effects and therefore induce dry mouth, blurred vision, urinary retention and constipation. Many also induce sedation, but this is turned to advantage in that such drugs then have added usefulness in the treatment of agitated, depressed patients. The stimulant action of antidepressant drugs may also result in insomnia and convulsions, although this is rare at normal doses; antidepressants should be used with caution by those who suffer from epilepsy.

A newer form of antidepressant agent is mirtazapine (Zispin®), which is an antagonist of α_2-adrenoceptors; the actions of this drug are in line with the monoamine theory as it would be expected to increase the release of noradrenaline at the synapse.

One of the major downfalls of the monoamine hypothesis of depression is the fact that all of the antidepressant agents produce their biochemical effects, for example re-uptake inhibition, within hours of administration, but the clinical effects normally take 2 weeks to become apparent. The reason for this discrepancy in the time course of effects is still unknown, despite being recognised for over 30 years.

■ 3.3.2 DRUGS USED IN THE TREATMENT OF NEURODEGENERATIVE DISORDERS

With the increased ability of medicine to prevent illness and to decrease the consequences of illness, people can expect to live longer, and to remain active well into old age. This is generally seen as a positive benefit of modern medicine, but one consequence has been an increase in the incidence and prevalence of neurodegenerative disorders such as Parkinson's disease and Alzheimer's disease. Such disorders are not typically considered to be 'psychiatric disorders', but because of the obvious involvement of CNS biochemistry in their aetiology and the potential for the use of drugs acting on the CNS in their treatment, it is appropriate to describe the drugs used within this chapter.

3.3.2.1 Parkinson's disease

Parkinson's disease develops in approximately 1 per 500 of the population, with the onset of disease occurring after the age of 50 in two-thirds of cases. The disease may be a consequence of the ageing process, which is true Parkinson's disease, or it may be a consequence of head injury, infection such as encephalitis or of some drug treatments; in these latter incidences the condition is more normally referred to as parkinsonism. The symptoms of parkinsonism concern movement, thus there is a resting tremor, which decreases during voluntary activity. As the disease progresses there is muscle rigidity with decreased voluntary movement. The decreased movement affects not only the limbs but also the face, the sufferers therefore exhibit a lack of emotion, which may not represent their true feelings, and have problems such as dribbling and difficulties with feeding.

Dopamine is not able
to penetrate the blood–
brain barrier but ʟ-dopa
readily crosses the
blood–brain barrier
and is subsequently
metabolised to dopamine

Post-mortem studies indicate that parkinsonism is associated with reduced function of the dopaminergic neurones of the basal ganglia, most notably the nigro-striatal pathway, the treatments for the condition therefore seek to restore dopaminergic function. The most obvious approach to resolve this problem would be to administer dopamine; unfortunately this is not possible because dopamine is not able to penetrate the blood–

brain barrier (see Chapter 10). The natural precursor of dopamine is the amino acid dihydroxyphenylalanine (levodopa or L-dopa) which is readily able to cross the blood–brain barrier and is subsequently metabolised to dopamine by L-amino acid decarboxylase. The most common therapy for the treatment of parkinsonism is thus administration of L-dopa. Because L-amino acid decarboxylase is also present in the periphery, however, a significant proportion of the administered L-dopa is converted to dopamine and subsequently to noradrenaline outside of the brain. This not only reduces the bioavailability of the administered L-dopa but also gives rise to a number of side-effects such as tachycardia, arrhythmias, nausea and vomiting. This problem can be overcome by the co-administration of a peripheral decarboxylase inhibitor – a drug that inhibits the conversion of L-dopa to dopamine but does not cross the blood–brain barrier.

Treatment with L-dopa together with a peripheral decarboxylase inhibitor usually brings an improvement of the symptoms for 3–5 years, after which the condition again begins to worsen. The reason for this limitation in the effectiveness of L-dopa is not fully understood but may reflect the further degeneration of dopaminergic neurones of the basal ganglia. It is these neurones that possess the enzyme required for the conversion of the L-dopa to dopamine. Some patients also experience an 'on–off effect' of the L-dopa in which the symptoms suddenly deteriorate, without apparent reason. Further adminstration of the L-dopa is required to regain control of the symptoms. Other adverse effects of L-dopa include involuntary movements and hallucinations (see later), although these usually subside if the dose is decreased.

Another approach to the treatment of parkinsonism is the administration of an inhibitor of the subtype of monoamine oxidase responsible for the breakdown of dopamine – monoamine oxidase B. Selegiline is a selective inhibitor of MAO B which can be used alone in the treatment of early parkinsonism, or more usually used in combination with L-dopa in the treatment of more advanced stages of the disorder. Other treatments include amantidine, which causes the release of presynaptic dopamine, and the dopamine receptor agonists bromocriptine and apomorphine. The advantage of the latter two agents is that they do not require functioning dopaminergic neurones for their actions.

Another approach to the relief of parkinsonism is the use of anticholinergic (antimuscarinic) agents. Anticholinergic agents cause constipation, urinary retention and decreased salivation, and some sources state that these agents were initially used in parkinsonism to facilitate the care of the patients who suffer problems of incontinence and dribbling. These agents do, however, improve the motor deficits. The mechanism of action of these agents is unclear, but it is known that increased dopamine activity in the basal ganglia is associated with decreased cholinergic activity in other brain areas, thus an alternative to increasing dopaminergic function appears to be reducing cholinergic function.

As described in Section 3.2.7, dopamine also plays a role in the aetiology of schizophrenia. Schizophrenia has been associated with an increase in dopaminergic function and is treated with dopamine antagonists, whereas parkinsonism is associated with decreased dopaminergic function and is treated with dopamine agonists. Although these two disorders probably arise in different brain areas, the former in the midbrain/limbic system and the latter in the basal ganglia, there is some interaction. For example, administration of L-dopa for the relief of parkinsonism has been seen to induce hallucinations in some patients; a symptom of schizophrenia. Treatment of schizophrenia with a dopamine antagonist, on the other hand, is associated with the onset of extrapyramidal side-effects, the symptoms of which are involuntary tremor and muscle rigidity: parkinsonism. In the case of the adverse psychological effects of L-dopa, the problem can usually be overcome

Sufferers of Parkinson's disease may have the problems of incontinence and dribbling: anticholinergic agents cause constipation, urinary retention and decreased salivation

by a decrease in dose, but decreasing the dose of the antipsychotic medication in an attempt to alleviate the extrapyramidal symptoms usually results in reappearance of the psychosis.

The extrapyramidal side-effects of antipsychotic agents cannot be prevented by administration of L-dopa or a dopamine antagonist because the two treatments are obviously incompatible. The only remedy, therefore, is to co-administer an anticholinergic agent. Such drugs reduce the severity of the extrapyramidal side-effects without impinging on the psychological symptoms. Paradoxically it is the anticholinergic 'side-effects' of the antipsychotic agent chlorpromazine that confer upon it advantages over the more selective dopamine antagonist haloperidol in terms of the likelihood of inducing extrapyramidal effects.

3.3.2.2 Huntington's chorea

Huntington's chorea is an inherited disorder characterised by severe involuntary jerky movements and dementia; chorea means 'dance', as in choreographer. It is believed that the disorder may be associated with a reduction in GABA function, possibly with increased dopaminergic function. The drugs used for the relief of the symptoms of Huntington's disease are therefore dopamine antagonists such as chlorpromazine and the other antipsychotic agents, and a drug that depletes dopamine stores, tetrabenazine. GABA agonists such as baclofen, and drugs that enhance GABA function, for example benzodiazepines and barbiturates, may also be of use.

3.3.2.3 Alzheimer's disease

Alzheimer's disease is a condition in which there is progressive loss of cognitive function in the absence of any other form of brain insult such as drug toxicity or head injury. It is generally seen to be related to age, thus 5% of 65-year-olds suffer from Alzheimer's disease, but at 95 years of age the prevalence is approximately 90%, to some degree. Because of the increasing mean age of the population, and the percentage of the population that are now over the age of 65, the cause of Alzheimer's disease has been the focus of extensive research, and many advances have been made. The most influential finding to date has been the identification of reduced acetylcholine, choline acetyl transferase and nicotinic receptors in post-mortem brains from Alzheimer sufferers. The aim of therapies is to increase cholinergic function in the brain, this has led to the introduction of inhibitors of cholinesterase such as donepezil (Aricept®) and rivastigmine (Exelon®), which have both been shown to have some beneficial effect in these patients. Interestingly, it has also been observed that cigarette smokers may obtain some protection against Alzheimer's disease, probably because of the enhanced nicotinic activity.

■ 3.4 DRUG DEPENDENCE AND SUBSTANCE ABUSE

The use of drugs for recreational, non-medical purposes is very common. In a recent (1998) study in the UK, 48% of a sample of male and 44% of a sample of female university undergraduates reported ever having used cannabis, with 2% of the males and 6% of the females using it weekly. In the same cohort, 7% of the males and 10% of the females reported having used amphetamines, whereas 5% of the males and 7% of the females reported having used ecstasy.

In a sample of slightly older subjects, junior hospital doctors, 64% of the males and 57% of the females reported ever having used cannabis; approximately 30% of the subjects were using cannabis at the time of the survey. Approximately 10% of the doctors reported current use of amphetamines, cocaine, amyl nitrate or ecstasy.

The effects and mechanisms of action of potential drugs of abuse such as the ben-zodiazepines and the opioids have been described earlier in this chapter (Sections 3.2.2–3.2.5), the actions of ecstasy, amphetamine, cocaine, LSD and cannabis will be described here.

■ 3.4.1 THE ACTIONS OF ECSTASY

Ecstasy (MDMA; 3,4-methylene-dioxymethamphetamine) is classed as a hallucinogen. Users report increased feeling of elation, agreeableness, energy and mental confusion, other effects include increased heart rate, increased body temperature, sweating, dehyd-ration, dilated pupils and tight jaw. There may also be auditory or visual hallucinations with impaired perceptions, 'enhanced insight' and impaired judgement. The nature of the effects ('trip') are not dose dependent but are influenced by the environment, and 'flashbacks' of trips may occur during drug-free days.

Ecstasy acts in a way similar to amphetamine (see Section 3.4.2) in that it causes the release of the neurotransmitters noradrenaline, dopamine and 5-HT from nerve ter-minals and has agonist effects at 5-HT receptors. These actions account for the stimulant effects in the CNS and the sympathomimetic actions such as tachycardia; the agonist effects at the 5-HT receptors are responsible for the hallucinatory effects.

Chemical variation of the core MDMA molecule leads to the production of novel drugs, with similar pharmacological actions. Theses novel agents are known as designer drugs, some of which are not yet covered by current legislation.

■ 3.4.2 THE ACTIONS OF AMPHETAMINE

Amphetamine is structurally related to the catecholamine neurotransmitters noradrenaline and dopamine, it acts in the CNS to cause the release of noradrenaline and dopamine from nerve terminals. The effects of amphetamine and derivatives such as methamphetamine are mediated mainly by the release of stored dopamine.

Users of amphetamines report feelings of increased alertness, elation, a feeling of well-being, increased competence and heightened sexual experiences. There have also been reports of stereotypy in humans, a phenomenon in which the individual repeatedly performs purposeless actions such as signing their name or brushing their hair. In the periphery, high doses of amphetamine cause tachycardia, hypertension and possible cardiovascular collapse.

As the effects of the amphetamine subside the user 'crashes', with feelings of dysphoria, tiredness, irritability and depression; continued periods of use result in exhaustion. Amphetamines do not induce physical dependence, but there is psychological depend-ence, with abstinence resulting in fatigue and depression. It has been suggested that long-term use of amphetamines may result in personality changes, delusions, paranoia and psychosis, a suggestion supported by the fact that chronic amphetamine treatment in rats has been used as a model of schizophrenia.

Users are unable to differentiate the effects of cocaine from those of amphetamine

■ 3.4.3 THE ACTIONS OF COCAINE

Users are unable to differentiate the effects of cocaine from those of amphetamine, except that cocaine has a much shorter duration of action (30 minutes). The mechanism of action of cocaine differs from that of amphetamine, however: cocaine increases dopaminergic function by preventing its re-uptake (inactivation) rather than by inducing its release.

Freebase ('crack') cocaine is more rapidly absorbed than the hydrochloride salt and can be inhaled (smoked). This rapid absorption produces a more intense 'rush', but is followed by a 'crash'.

■ 3.4.4 THE ACTIONS OF LSD

LSD (lysergic acid diethylamide), like mescaline and psilocybin (magic mushrooms) is chemically related to the neurotransmitter 5-HT. In humans it acts as an agonist at 5-HT receptors, but by negative feedback it reduces total 5-HT activity. As is the case for ecstasy (Section 3.4.1), this action on 5-HT receptors results in altered perceptions and hallucinations. Users report seeing familiar objects and people as brighly coloured and distorted, and the senses become confused, such that sounds are perceived as colours. There may also be 'out of body' experiences where the user is able to 'look down upon themselves and observe their own bizarre behaviour'. Occasionally bad 'trips' may result in suicide or murder. These bad 'trips' may be long lasting, and a single dose may precipitate psychosis. Interestingly, animals will not self-administer LSD, indicating that they find its effects aversive. Rapid tolerance develops to LSD, but there are no withdrawal effects.

■ 3.4.5 THE ACTIONS OF CANNABIS

Cannabis is obtained from hemp, *Cannabis sativa*, the dried leaf of the hemp is marijuana, the extract (resin) is hashish. The active component of cannabis is D^1-tetrahydrocannabinol (THC). THC acts on specific G-protein coupled (G_i) receptors in the brain to cause mood lability (from euphoria to anxiety), heightened perception (colour, music, smell, etc.). THC may also cause impaired judgement and drowsiness. The presence of a cannabinoid receptor also raises the question of the possible existence of a possible endogenous cannabinoid transmitter. There is little evidence of tolerance or dependence to THC; however, withdrawal may cause nausea, agitation, irritability and confusion. It is relatively non-toxic (except that it is smoked with tobacco), but in rats it is teratogenic.

There has been much debate about the legalisation of cannabis in the UK, and its potential beneficial effects in the relief of nausea and as a palliative in terminal illness, but as yet, unlike some other European countries, cannabis use in the UK remains an offence.

■ SUMMARY

- In general terms, drugs act on the central nervous system (CNS) to influence the balance of excitatory and inhibitory activity, thus drugs used to induce sleep or prevent 'over-activity' of the brain (for example convulsions) act by enhancing the actions of inhibitory neurotransmitters or decreasing the activity of excitatory neurotransmitters. Drugs used to treat conditions associated with 'under-activity' of the brain, for example depression, act by enhancing the activity of excitatory neurotransmitters or decreasing the actions of inhibitory neurotransmitters.
- Gaseous and vapour general anaesthetics act either by dissolving into the nerve cell membrane and disrupting the activity of the cell (the lipid theory) or by interacting with proteins associated with the cell membrane, for example ion channels and receptors (the protein theory). Intravenous general anaesthetics act on defined membrane-bound receptors to decrease cellular activity.
- The narcotic analgesics such as morphine and heroin mimic the body's own endorphins and act on specific opioid receptors to relieve pain. The actions of these drugs on opioid receptors elsewhere in the body are responsible for other effects of these drugs, for example antidiarrhoeal, cough suppressant, etc.
- Anticonvulsant agents produce their effects either by enhancing the effects of the inhibitory neurotransmitter GABA or by stabilising the neuronal membrane. Anxiolytic and hypnotic agents, similarly, enhance the effects of GABA.

- The drugs used to treat psychoses appear to act by antagonism of the dopamine receptor, although some of these agents also have effects on 5-HT receptors. Antipsychotic agents are effective in the treatment of disorders such as schizophrenia but precipitate a large number of adverse effects, due to effects on receptors other than dopamine receptors. The main adverse effects of the antipsychotic agents, however, are a direct consequence of antagonism of dopamine receptors in the extrapyramidal system of the brain.

- Antidepressant agents increase neuronal activity either by preventing the metabolism of the neurotransmitters 5-HT and noradrenaline, or by preventing their inactivation by re-uptake into the nerve terminal. Some agents are selective inhibitors of either 5-HT or noradrenaline, but there appears to be little advantage in terms of efficacy.

- Degenerative diseases of the central nervous system are treated effectively by administration of precursors of the appropriate neurotransmitter, or by prevention of neurotransmitter inactivation.

- Because drugs that act on the central nervous system have the potential to alter mood, they also have the potential for misuse. Problems of drug misuse arise not only from the physical effects of the drugs but also because of the tendency to cause tolerance and dependence.

■ REVISION QUESTIONS

For each question select the most appropriate answer. Correct answers are presented in Appendix 1.

1. Which of the following responses are *not* induced by morphine:
   (a) suppression of pain;
   (b) inhibition of gastrointestinal motility;
   (c) cough;
   (d) sedation;
   (e) euphoria.

2. Which of the following explains the anticonvulsant effects of sodium valproate:
   (a) antagonism of the $GABA_A$ receptor;
   (b) stimulation of the benzodiazepine receptor;
   (c) activation of a chloride ion channel;
   (d) blockade of voltage-gated sodium ion channels;
   (e) blockade of a voltage-gated potassium ion channel.

3. Which of the following explains the anxiolytic effects of diazepam:
   (a) antagonism of the $GABA_A$ receptor;
   (b) stimulation of the $GABA_A$ receptor;
   (c) opening of a ligand-gated chloride ion channel;
   (d) opening of ligand-gated sodium ion channels;
   (e) blockade of a voltage-gated potassium ion channel.

4. Which of the following is *not* a potential adverse effect of the antipsychotic agent chlorpromazine:
   (a) extrapyramidal side-effects;
   (b) excess secretion of prolactin;
   (c) anticholinergic effects;
   (d) hypertension;
   (e) tardive dyskinesia.

5. Which of the following groups of drugs would be unlikely to exhibit any antidepressant activity:

    (a) monoamine oxidase inhibitors;

    (b) decarboxylase inhibitors;

    (c) non-selective monoamine re-uptake inhibitors;

    (d) selective inhibitors of serotonin re-uptake;

    (e) selective inhibitors of noradrenaline re-uptake.

6. A deficiency of which of the following neurotransmitters is believed to be involved in the aetiology of Alzheimer's disease:

    (a) acetylcholine;

    (b) noradrenaline;

    (c) serotonin;

    (d) dopamine;

    (e) GABA.

■ SELECTED READING

Frazer, A. and Morilak, Q.A. (1998) Drugs for the treatment of affective (mood) disorders. In Brody, T.M., Larner, J. and Minneman, K.P. (eds) *Human Pharmacology: Molecular to Clinical* (Third edition), (St. Louis: Mosby), 349–363.

Galbraith, A., Bullock, S., Manias, E., Hunt, B. and Richards, A. (1999) Section VII Drugs to alter behaviour and motor activity. In Galbraith, A., Bullock, S., Manias, E., Hunt, B. and Richards, A. *Fundamentals of Pharmacology*, (Harlow: Addison Wesley Longman), 257–321.

Galbraith, A., Bullock, S., Manias, E., Hunt, B. and Richards, A. (1999) Section VIII Drugs used to relieve pain and produce anaesthesia. In Galbraith, A., Bullock, S., Manias, E., Hunt, B. and Richards, A. *Fundamentals of Pharmacology*, (Harlow: Addison Wesley Longman), 323–366.

Gudelsky, G.A. (1998) Antipsychotic agents. In Brody, T.M., Larner, J. and Minneman, K.P. (eds) *Human Pharmacology: Molecular to Clinical* (Third edition), (St. Louis: Mosby), 339–348.

Holtzman, S.G. and Yung-Fong, S. (1998) Pain control with opioid analgesics. In Brody, T.M., Larner, J. and Minneman, K.P. (eds) *Human Pharmacology: Molecular to Clinical* (Third edition), (St. Louis: Mosby), 395–408.

Rang, H.P., Dale, M.M. and Ritter, J.M. (1999) Section 4: The Central Nervous System. In Rang, H.P., Dale, M.M. and Ritter, J.M. *Pharmacology* (Fourth edition), (Edinburgh: Churchill Livingstone), 464–633.

Rech, R.H. (1998) Drugs used to treat anxiety and related disorders. In Brody, T.M., Larner, J. and Minneman, K.P. (eds) *Human Pharmacology: Molecular to Clinical* (Third edition), (St. Louis: Mosby), 365–372.

Stringer, J.L. (1998) Drugs for seizure disorders (Epilepsies). In Brody, T.M., Larner, J. and Minneman, K.P. (eds) *Human Pharmacology: Molecular to Clinical* (Third edition), (St. Louis: Mosby), 373–383.

Yung-Fong, S. and Holtzman, S.G. (1998) Pain control with general anaesthetics. In Brody, T.M., Larner, J. and Minneman, K.P. (eds) *Human Pharmacology: Molecular to Clinical* (Third edition), (St. Louis: Mosby), 421–434.

■ COMPUTER-AIDED LEARNING PACKAGES

Further details of these learning packages can be found at
http://www.coacs.com/PCCAL/
and
http://cbl.leeds.ac.uk/raven/pha/phCAL.html

Basic Psychopharmacology (version 2.0), Pharmacy Consortium for Computer Aided Learning (PCCAL), COACS Ltd, University of Bath.

Drug Dependence (version 1.96), Pharma-CAL-ogy, British Pharmacological Society, University of Leeds.

Epilepsy (version 2.0), Pharmacy Consortium for Computer Aided Learning (PCCAL), COACS Ltd, University of Bath.

Movement Disorders (version 1.96), Pharma-CAL-ogy, British Pharmacological Society, University of Leeds.

Schizophrenia (version 1.96), Pharma-CAL-ogy, British Pharmacological Society, University of Leeds.

THE TREATMENT OF CARDIOVASCULAR DISORDERS

■ 4.1 INTRODUCTION

The cardiovascular system comprises the heart and the blood vessels, its function is to transport blood, at the appropriate pressure, to all areas of the body. This function is achieved by the constant but variable activity of the heart, which beats approximately 3 billion times during the average lifetime, together with a vasculature of adjustable capacity. Together the heart and vasculature must provide a blood supply which is responsive to the needs of the tissues, thus the activity of the heart increases as the body's demand for oxygen increases and the vasculature contracts or dilates to direct blood flow to the areas of greatest need. The ability of the cardiovascular system to perform its function can be compromised by a failure at any point of the system, for example failure of the heart to contract rhythmically or with sufficient force, blockage of a blood vessel or inability of a blood vessel to constrict or dilate appropriately. Cardiovascular disease is the most common cause of death in the developed world, and is a major cause of disability; it is because of this that the development and use of drugs to treat or prevent cardiovascular disease has achieved such prominence in pharmacology and medicine.

Cardiovascular disease is the most common cause of death in the developed world; it is because of this that the development of drugs to treat or prevent cardiovascular disease has achieved such prominence

This chapter will describe the actions and properties of those drugs that alter the activity of the cardiovascular system by effects on the heart or the vasculature; drugs that alter cardiovascular function indirectly, such as those acting on the kidney and the blood, are covered elsewhere (see Chapter 5).

■ 4.2 ESSENTIAL PHYSIOLOGY OF THE CARDIOVASCULAR SYSTEM

Before considering disorders of the cardiovascular system and the use of drugs in their treatment, it is important to understand its normal physiology. It is beyond the scope of this text to review the physiology of the cardiovascular system comprehensively, the reader is therefore referred to textbooks of physiology; however, those features that must be appreciated before the actions of drugs can be understood will be described. The basic physiology of the cardiovascular system will be described in two sections: first the physiology of the heart, and secondly the physiology of the vasculature.

■ 4.2.1 THE HEART

Cardiac muscle cells are similar to those of other excitable tissues such as nerves and muscles in that they possess ion channels within their cell membrane and are therefore able to depolarise and repolarise. Under normal resting conditions the ventricular muscle cells have a resting potential of 60–80mV across the membrane, with the inside of the cell being negative with respect to the outside. Like other excitable tissues, if the membrane potential of cardiac cells moves towards zero (i.e. depolarises), voltage-gated sodium channels open briefly to allow rapid influx of sodium ions, resulting in a shift of the membrane potential to approximately +20mV. The sodium ion channels are only open briefly, thus as they close the membrane potential of the cell begins to return to a negative value, primarily because of the opening of potassium channels. Unlike non-cardiac excitable membranes, however, repolarisation is delayed by the slow opening and closing of L-type calcium channels, which allow calcium ions to enter the cell. The activity of these calcium channels has the effect of maintaining the membrane potential at a value of about −10mV: the plateau phase. As the calcium channels close, the membrane potential moves towards −20mV and potassium channels begin to open slowly, enabling efflux of potassium ions and the repolarisation of the cell to its original resting potential. Cardiac cells therefore differ from other excitable cells in that following the initial depolarisation and partial repolarisation there is a plateau phase when the membrane potential is small and the cell is relatively refractory to further depolarisation.

The influx of calcium into the cardiac muscle cells during the plateau phase of repolarisation, together with release of calcium from intracellular stores, results in contraction of the cardiac muscle. The specialised conducting tissues ensure that the heart muscle contracts in an ordered manner, with the atria contracting prior to the ventricles. Furthermore, the long refractory period ensures that the cardiac muscle must relax fully before it again contracts. The rhythmic contraction of the heart, in an orderly manner, enables it to function efficiently as a pump. This orderly activity is a direct consequence of the nature of the ion channels of cardiac tissue and the presence of specialised conducting tissue.

The other important feature of cardiac tissue is that there are groups of cells within the muscle which spontaneously depolarise; they do not require the depolarisation of adjacent cells to induce voltage-gated sodium channel opening. These cells are called pacemaker cells. Pacemaker cells spontaneously depolarise because they possess ion channels which allow a slow, but constant influx of ions (leakage), this in turn causes slow, but steady, depolarisation, ultimately resulting in opening calcium channels (these cells lack the normal voltage-gated sodium channels); it is the activity of these calcium channels that results in the depolarisation of the pacemaker cell. There are several groups of pacemaker cells, the most important being the sino-atrial node and the atrio-ventricular node. Each group of pacemaker cells spontaneously depolarises at slightly different rates, but because of the existence of specialised conducting tissue within the heart, the action potential arising from one group of pacemaker cells is rapidly conducted to other groups, causing their premature depolarisation. It can therefore be seen that the first pacemaker to depolarise initiates the depolarisation of the whole tissue, and is thus the pacemaker for the whole heart.

■ 4.2.2 THE VASCULATURE

The function of the vasculature is to transport blood to all tissues in order to supply oxygen and nutrients and to remove carbon dioxide and other metabolic waste products. The blood is also important for heat distribution and temperature regulation. In order for the blood to be able to perform its functions it must be supplied at an appropriate pressure. Blood vessels therefore need to be able to direct the flow of blood to those organs where the demand is greatest, to maintain appropriate pressures under a range of physiological conditions, and to permit free exchange of gases, fluid and solutes.

Blood vessels can be divided into five separate classes: arteries, arterioles, capillaries, venules and veins. Arteries and arterioles have thick, smooth-muscle walls with elastic properties. The elastic properties are important in the dampening of the blood pressure surges resulting from the pulsatile nature of the cardiac output. Constriction of arteries and arterioles is also important in directing blood flow and the control of blood pressure. The capillaries are leaky, thin-walled, narrow vessels through which there is relatively unhindered exchange of fluids and solutes; the degree of fluid and solute exchange through capillaries is dependent upon the pressure of blood within them. The primary function of the venules and veins is to transport the deoxygenated blood back to the heart. Venoconstriction, however, has the effect of increasing the blood pressure within the capillaries, thus increasing the movement of fluids into the tissues, and of increasing the pressure of the blood returning to the heart (venous return), which increases cardiac output. It can therefore be seen that the venules and veins are also important in maintaining the functional efficiency of the cardiovascular system.

Multiple factors are co-ordinated in the control of blood pressure, as stated in Chapter 2, the most important of these is the activity of the autonomic nervous system. The autonomic system monitors blood pressure by means of baroreceptors in the aortic arch and the carotid sinus. A decrease in blood pressure leads to a decrease in parasympathetic activity and an increase in sympathetic activity. This results in increased rate and force of cardiac contraction and vasoconstriction, thus causing an increase in blood pressure. Increased blood pressure results in increased parasympathetic activity and decreased sympathetic activity. Similar responses are produced when chemosensors in the aortic arch, carotid sinus or brainstem detect a decrease in the oxygen content of the blood. The autonomic nervous system, including the adrenal medulla, therefore modulates blood pressure in response to the demands of the whole body, for example at times of exercise or stress.

More local control of blood flow and pressure is achieved by the release of autocoids (local hormones) and other mediators, such as serotonin (5-HT) and histamine, for example as part of the inflammatory process (see Chapter 9). The cellular lining of the blood vessels, the endothelium, is also important in the control of local blood pressure. Mediators known to be released by the endothelium include prostaglandins, nitric oxide and endothelins; the endothelium also possesses a complete renin–angiotensin system (see Chapter 5). Prostaglandin I_2 (prostacyclin) and PGE_2 induce vasodilation; the latter also inhibits noradrenaline release from sympathetic nerve terminals, thus further inhibiting vasoconstriction. PGG_2 and PGH_2 act on thromboxane receptors (see Chapter 9) to cause vasoconstriction. Nitric oxide, formerly called endothelial derived relaxing factor (EDRF), causes vascular relaxation by inducing production of cyclic GMP (see Chapter 1); nitric oxide itself acts as a second messenger for substances such as bradykinin and acetylcholine. The presence of the renin–angiotensin system, specifically angiotensin-converting enzyme, within the endothelium further allows for local vasoconstriction, thus inducing local increases in blood pressure.

■ 4.3 DISORDERS OF CARDIAC RHYTHM AND THEIR TREATMENT

The generation of the cardiac action potential and its conduction are described in Section 4.2.1. Any abnormality of the normal rhythmic contraction of the heart is called arrhythmia or dysrhythmia. Arrhythmias may occur for a variety or reasons. Any disruption of the ability of the specialised tissues to conduct the action potential around the heart will influence cardiac rhythm. Thus damage due to local anoxia, for example, may result in the impulse generated by the sino-atrial node being unable to travel to the ventricles. In this circumstance, 'heart block', the atria contract with a normal rhythm, but the ventricles contract at a slower inherent rhythm. Arrhythmia may also occur when electrical conductivity is delayed, such that the action potential is able to re-depolarise some cells which have passed through the refractory period. Other forms of arrhythmia, such as ectopic beats and fibrillation, occur when cells that are not normally pacemakers spontaneously depolarise, for example due to premature opening of voltage-gated sodium channels. These cells then take on the role of pacemaker cells, resulting in uncoordinated waves of contraction in different areas of the heart. Such abnormal pacemaker activity may occur following disruption of the local ionic environment, for example increased intracellular calcium, or excessive stimulation by catecholamines.

Arrhythmias may occur following disruption of the local ionic environment, for example increased intracellular calcium, or excessive stimulation by catecholamines

Several classes of drugs are available for the treatment and prevention of arrhythmias, most of these act by blocking cardiac sodium, potassium or calcium ion channels. An important feature of these antiarrhythmic drugs, however, is that they seem to act selectively on damaged tissue, or tissues that are depolarising at abnormally rapid rates. The overall effect is that these drugs act on cells to decrease the rate of depolarisation or repolarisation, thus decreasing that rate at which the cells can repeatedly depolarise. Because the cardiac cells normally have a long refractory period, it can be seen why antiarrhythmic drugs have little or no effect on normally functioning pacemaker cells, but inhibit the activity of rapidly, spontaneously depolarising cells. The antiarrhythmic drugs will be discussed under four headings: sodium channel blockers, β-adrenoceptor antagonists, potassium channel blockers and calcium channel blockers, although a separate notation, the Vaughan Williams classification, will also be indicated.

■ 4.3.1 SODIUM CHANNEL BLOCKERS (VAUGHAN WILLIAMS CLASS I)

Antiarrhythmic drugs which block sodium ion channels have traditionally been called 'class I antiarrhythmics'. These drugs, for example quinidine, procainamide and lignocaine (lidocaine) (see Box 4.1), act in a manner similar to that of local anaesthetics, and therefore depress the activity of the cardiac cells without influencing the pacemaker cells. As described above, the effect is frequency dependent, meaning that rapidly depolarising cells are more affected by the drugs than normally depolarising ones. The overall effect of these drugs is to decrease the rate at which ectopic (abnormal) pacemaker cells depolarise, thus re-asserting the dominance of the natural pacemakers. The drugs also decrease the speed at which the cardiac myocytes can depolarise, thus decreasing an accelerated rate of contraction.

An important feature of antiarrhythmic drugs is that they seem to act selectively on tissues that are depolarising at abnormally rapid rates

These drugs are used particularly when the arrhythmia affects both the atria and the ventricles. Some members of this group, for example quinidine and flecainide, have enhanced activity because of additional actions; in the case of the former, blockade of potassium channels and in the case of flecainide, β-adrenoceptor antagonist effects.

■ 4.3.2 β-ADRENOCEPTOR ANTAGONISTS (VAUGHAN WILLIAMS CLASS II)

The effects of the archetypal β-adrenoceptor antagonist, propranolol, are dependent, first, on its receptor-mediated effect and, secondly, on its ability, at high concentrations, to block sodium ion channels. This latter action, the 'quinidine-like effect' explains a large proportion of its antiarrhythmic properties, but receptor blockade is also important. By reducing the effects of the endogenous catecholamines on the sino-atrial node,

■ *Box 4.1* Properties and actions of agents used for the treatment of arrhythmias

Drug class	Agent	Proprietary name
Sodium channel blockers	Quinidine	Kinidin Durules®
	Procainamide	Pronestyl®
	Lignocaine (lidocaine)	Xylocard®
	Flecainide	Tambocor®
β-Adrenoceptor antagonists	Esmolol	Brevibloc®
Potassium channel blockers	Amiodarone	Cordarone X®
	Sotalol	Beta-Cardone®
Calcium channel blockers	Verapamil	Cordilox®

β-adrenoceptor antagonists are able to slow the rate of depolarisation of pacemaker cells (see Chapter 2). Examples of the β-adrenoceptor antagonists used for the treatment of arrhythmias are presented in Box 4.1.

■ **4.3.3 POTASSIUM CHANNEL BLOCKERS (VAUGHAN WILLIAMS CLASS III)**

The three drugs of this class are bretylium, amiodarone and sotalol. Bretylium reduces the arrhythmia by prolonging the duration of the action potential and the refractory period. This is achieved partially by blockade of potassium channels, and partially by inhibition of noradrenaline release. The latter action has the effect of slowing the rate of depolarisation of the pacemaker cells. Amiodarone also blocks potassium channels, but also blocks sodium and calcium channels and is a β-adrenoceptor antagonist. It is unclear which of these actions is primarily responsible for its antiarrhythmic effect. The final drug, sotalol, is a β-adrenoceptor antagonist, but it also has potassium channel blocking properties; this latter property is probably responsible for its efficacy.

■ **4.3.4 CALCIUM CHANNEL BLOCKERS (VAUGHAN WILLIAMS CLASS IV)**

Calcium channel blockers are only active against the L (long-lasting, large)-type calcium channels. Several calcium channel blockers are available (see Section 4.7.5), but only verapamil and diltiazem (see Box 4.1) are effective against cardiac calcium channels, probably because there are several different subtypes of the L-type calcium channel. These two drugs have the effect of decreasing the influx of calcium into the pacemaker cell, thus slowing natural pacemaker activity, and also blocking calcium channels in cardiac myocytes. The latter effect means that the cardiac myocytes repolarise more rapidly because the calcium channels are unable to produce the plateau effect on the membrane potential (see Section 4.2.1) and, because less calcium is available for the process of muscle contraction, the rate and force of cardiac contraction is reduced.

Because calcium channel blockers also have effects on the vasculature, their use in the treatment of arrhythmias can cause a decrease in blood pressure (see Section 4.7.5), resulting in a reflex tachycardia. This increase in heart rate may exacerbate the arrhythmia.

Calcium channel blockers are only active against the L (long-lasting, large)-type calcium channels. These drugs have the effect of decreasing the influx of calcium into the pacemaker cell, thus slowing natural pacemaker activity, and also blocking calcium channels in cardiac myocytes

■ **4.4 HEART FAILURE AND ITS TREATMENT**

If the ability of the left ventricle to contract (or relax) is lost, its function as a pump is compromised. The ensuing effect is to deprive the tissues of nutrients and oxygen, causing organ failure, giving rise to a multitude of symptoms; this is heart failure. Because of the homeostatic processes in place, for example vasoconstriction and sodium retention, heart failure does not initially cause a decrease in arterial blood pressure; however, there is an increase of back-pressure in the veins because blood is unable to pass through the heart at an appropriate rate. Unfortunately the homeostatic mechanisms themselves increase peripheral resistance and thus place further strain on the failing heart. In many cases heart failure is symptomless because of the homeostasis, although because of the decreased cardiac reserve, deficiencies may become apparent at times of stress or exercise. As the condition worsens, the effects of the venous congestion increase, causing tissue and/or pulmonary oedema. It is because of this that the condition is often called congestive heart failure.

In many cases heart failure is symptomless, although deficiencies may become apparent at times of stress or exercise. As the condition worsens the effects of the venous congestion increase, causing tissue and/or pulmonary oedema: congestive heart failure

The aim of the drug therapies for heart failure is to increase cardiac output and blood perfusion of the organs. This is achieved by using drugs to increase the force of cardiac contraction or to reduce the peripheral resistance, thus reducing the load on the heart. Drugs may also be used to relieve the oedema and to prevent further changes in the cardiac tissue.

■ 4.4.1 CARDIAC GLYCOSIDES

Cardiac glycosides act directly on the heart to increase the force of contraction, they also slow the heart rate by an indirect effect (see later). The two most important cardiac glycosides are digoxin and digitoxin, which are present in the leaves of the foxglove (*Digitalis* sp.) and have been used for their effect on the heart for over 200 years (see Box 4.2). The cardiac glycosides produce their effects by inhibition of Na^+, K^+-ATPase. As stated in Section 4.2.1, cardiac muscle cells normally have a resting potential of approximately -60 to -80mV, this is achieved by the action of Na^+, K^+-ATPase, which pumps three sodium ions out of the cell in exchange for two potassium ions. By competing with potassium for binding to the enzyme, the cardiac glycosides inhibit the action of the pump and therefore reduce the resting membrane potential and increase the intracellular concentration of sodium. One consequence of the increased intracellular sodium concentration is a decreased sodium concentration gradient for a membrane-bound Na^+/Ca^{2+} pump which normally pumps calcium out of the cell by utilising the inward movement of sodium along the concentration gradient. The ultimate effect of the drugs is to increase intracellular calcium and, because calcium is essential for muscle contraction, to increase the extent of muscle contraction.

The effects of the cardiac glycosides, however, are not limited to the heart, thus Na^+, K^+-ATPase is inhibited at other sites around the body, especially in excitable tissues such as nerves. Cardiac glycosides have limited ability to cross the blood–brain barrier (see Chapter 10) but nerve cells of the autonomic nervous system are particularly susceptible to their effects. Because of these effects, the cardiac glycosides increase the release of acetylcholine from the vagus nerve, which leads to a decrease in heart rate, and increase the release of noradrenaline from sympathetic nerves, which results in vasoconstriction. One of these effects, the decreased heart rate, contributes markedly to the efficacy of these drugs in the relief of cardiac failure, by increasing the time available for filling of the ventricle during diastole, and therefore increasing cardiac output.

A major drawback to the use of cardiac glycosides in the treatment of cardiac failure is cardiotoxicity. At therapeutic doses, these drugs cause an increase in the force of contraction of the heart, and a decrease in heart rate. At slightly higher doses, however, the inhibition of the Na^+, K^+-ATPase results in a decreased transmembrane potential in cardiac cells, and therefore an increased excitability. This effect is manifested as an increased incidence of ventricular tachycardias and ventricular arrhythmias. The therapeutic index

■ *Box 4.2* Drugs used for the treatment of heart failure

Drug class	Agent	Proprietary name
Cardiac glycosides	Digoxin	Lanoxin®
Sympathomimetics	Dopamine	Select-A-Jet® Dopamine
	Dobutamine	Dobutrex®
		Posiject®
Phosphodiesterase inhibitors	Enoximone	Perfan®
	Milrinone	Primacor®

for cardiac glycosides is very low, thus as little as a 50% increase in dose can precipitate adverse events. The toxicity of cardiac glycosides can also be increased if plasma potassium concentrations fall, resulting in decreased competition for the Na^+,K^+-ATPase binding site. Reduced plasma potassium concentrations are a common feature of treatment with diuretic drugs, drugs which are commonly used to reduce the oedema associated with cardiac failure (see Chapter 5).

> The therapeutic index for cardiac glycosides is very low, thus as little as a 50% increase in dose can precipitate adverse events

■ 4.4.2 SYMPATHOMIMETICS

The only sympathomimetic agents used for the treatment of acute heart failure are dopamine and dobutamine (see Box 4.2). Both dopamine and dobutamine stimulate the β_1-adrenoceptors of the heart, which leads to an increase in intracellular calcium (see Chapter 2), the result of which is an increase in the force of contraction of the heart. Unfortunately, the sympathomimetics are also liable to cause increased heart rate and hypertension, which are deleterious; although dobutamine, which also has actions on β_2- and α-adrenoceptors, has less tendency to induce these effects.

■ 4.4.3 PHOSPHODIESTERASE INHIBITORS

Inhibitors of phosphodiesterase are known to reduce the degradation of cyclic nucleotides and therefore increase tissue concentrations of cAMP and cGMP (see Chapter 1). The heart, however, possesses a specific subtype of the enzyme called phosphodiesterase III, the inhibition of which results in an elevation of cAMP only. As cAMP is the second messenger for β_1-adrenoceptors in the heart, elevation of its concentrations by use of selective phosphospodiesterase III inhibitors such as enoximone and milrinone mimics the effects of β_1-adrenoceptor stimulation. These drugs are therefore useful for increasing the force of contraction of the heart in cardiac failure but, like the β_1-adrenoceptor agonists, carry with them the risk of tachycardia and arrhythmia; there is as yet no convincing clinical evidence that these drugs prolong survival in heart failure patients.

■ 4.4.4 VASODILATORS

Another method by which cardiac output can be increased is the reduction of peripheral resistance, although it is important that the resistance is not reduced so far as to reduce blood pressure. There are several drugs which are capable of reducing peripheral resistance, primarily by inducing peripheral dilatation. The mechanisms of action of these drugs include antagonism of the vascular α-adrenoceptors, blockade of vascular calcium channels and reduction of endogenous angiotensin activity. It is the latter drugs, angiotensin-converting enzyme (ACE) inhibitors, which have now become a mainstay of treatment for cardiac failure. Peripheral vasodilators are covered in detail in Section 4.7.6.

■ 4.4.5 DIURETICS

The final group of drugs used for the treatment of heart failure are diuretics. The drugs act via a variety of mechanisms to increase the excretion of fluid and solutes and therefore to decrease the volume of plasma and extracellular fluid. The mechanisms of action and therapeutic uses of diuretic drugs are described in Chapter 5. In the treatment of heart failure, diuretics such as the loop diuretics and the thiazide diutetics are beneficial because they reduce the work-load on the heart by decreasing the total plasma volume, and they decrease the extent of any pulmonary or peripheral oedema.

■ 4.5 DRUGS USED IN THE TREATMENT OF ANGINA

Angina is the severe chest pain, which often also spreads to the left arm and neck; it occurs when the heart is working under oxygen deficit. The oxygen deficiency is invariably caused by reduced blood flow to the cardiac muscle as a result of decreased competence of the coronary vessels due to atheroma. Three types of angina are recognised clinically: the first is stable angina, in which the pain occurs predictably at time of exertion, that is increased cardiac oxygen demand. The second type is unstable angina, this is where the pain onsets even with mild exertion and possibly even during rest. Unstable angina is due to fluctuations in the supply of oxygen to the cardiac tissues, usually due to blockage of the coronary vessels by platelet plaques, rather than changes in the demand. The final form of angina is variant angina, again this can occur at rest. Variant angina is caused by spasm of the coronary artery, causing cardiac ischaemia which is usually superimposed onto ischaemia due to atheroma. Variant angina in the absence of atheroma is known as Prinzmetal's disease. Treatments for angina aim to increase the supply of oxygen to the myocardium or to decrease the cardiac demand.

Angina may be treated with glyceryl trinitrate which is related to nitroglycerine, a component of dynamite

Stable angina may be treated with organic nitrates such as glyceryl trinitrate, isosorbide mononitrate or dinitrate or pentaerythritol tetranitrate (pentaerithrityl tetranitrate), see Box 4.3. These agents release nitric oxide (NO) which stimulates guanylyl cyclase to produce cyclic guanosine monophosphate (cGMP); the cGMP causes relaxation of the vascular smooth muscle. The dilation of the coronary arteries results in increased blood supply to the cardiac tissue, while dilation of other peripheral vessels lowers blood pressure

■ *Box 4.3* Mechanisms of action of drugs used in the relief of angina

Mechanism of action	Agent	Proprietary name
Nitric oxide donors	Glyceryl trinitrate	Nitromin®
		Nitro-Dur®
	Isosorbide dinitrate	Isordil®
	Isosorbide mononitrate	Mono-Cedocard®
	Pentaerythritol tetranitrate	Mycardol®
	(pentaerithrityl tetranitrate)	Brevibloc®
β-Adrenoceptor antagonists	Carvedilol	Eucardic®
	Nadolol	Corgard®
	Sotalol	Beta-Cardone®
Potassium channel activator	Nicorandil	Ikorel®
Calcium channel blockers	Diltiazem	Tildiem®

and decreases the work-load of the heart, this in turn decreases the oxygen demand by the cardiac muscle. These drugs may also be used in the treatment of variant angina and for the symptomatic relief of unstable angina.

Isosorbide and pentaerythritol are given orally, usually for the prophylaxis of angina; glyceryl trinitrate, when given sublingually, is more rapid in onset and therefore is of use for the relief of angina. The major side-effects of the organic nitrates relate to their primary mode of action, thus the vasodilation may cause headache and postural hypotension.

Another approach to the treatment of angina is the use of β-adrenoceptor antagonists. These act directly on the β_1-adrenoceptors of the heart to decrease the rate and force of contraction, thus decreasing oxygen demand. A potential risk, however, is an effect on the β_2-adrenoceptors of the coronary blood vessels, which may result in vasoconstriction. It is because of this latter effect that β-adrenoceptor antagonists are not used in the treatment of variant (Prinzmetal's) angina.

Calcium channel antagonists (see Sections 4.3.4 and 4.7.5) and potassium channel openers are also useful in the treatment of angina. Drugs such as verapamil and diltiazem act on L-type calcium channels to prevent the diffusion of calcium through the open channel. In the heart the result of this is to decrease the rate and force of contraction, while the vasodilation induced in the peripheral vasculature lowers blood pressure and cardiac work-load. Both actions reduce the oxygen demand of the cardiac tissue, and vasodilation of coronary vessels has the effect of increasing oxygen supply. Nicorandil both activates potassium channels and has a nitric oxide effect on guanylyl cyclase; both effects cause vasodilation and therefore relieve angina in a manner similar to that of the calcium channel antagonists.

At times of hypotension the obvious response is to decrease blood flow to non-essential organs while maintaining blood flow to organs such as the brain, heart and kidney. What actually happens, however, is an inappropriately increased flow of blood to the non-essential organs because of the accumulation of vasodilatory metabolites

■ 4.6 HYPOTENSION AND ITS TREATMENT

Severe hypotension is a medical emergency which often results in death. Causes of hypotension include haemorrhage, fluid loss of some other form (e.g. burns) and anaphylactic shock. At times of hypotension the homeostatic response is to decrease blood flow to non-essential organs while maintaining blood flow to organs such as the brain, heart and kidney. The accumulation of metabolic waste within the non-essential organs, however, usually results in local vasodilation which further reduces the systemic blood pressure. Many vasoactive drugs have been used to elevate abnormally low blood pressure, but the responses are often poor because of the multitude of mechanisms involved in the aetiology of the original hypotension. The most commonly used agents are the sympathomimetics such as adrenaline (epinephrine), noradrenaline (norepinephrine), dopamine and dobutamine which, to varying degrees, combine the properties of cardiac stimulation, α-adrenoceptor-mediated vasoconstriction and β-adrenoceptor-mediated vasodilation.

■ 4.7 HYPERTENSION AND ITS TREATMENT

Normal (average) systolic blood pressure is 120mmHg with a diastolic blood pressure of 80mmHg although these values usually increase with age. Increased blood pressure (hypertension) is known to be correlated with an increased risk of later disorders such as kidney failure, coronary thrombosis and stroke, which are collectively known as 'end organ damage', thus many millions of pounds are spent in an attempt to lower raised blood pressure; hypertension itself is symptomless. There is much dispute about the points at which antihypertensive therapy should be instituted and some clinicians believe that the diastolic blood pressure is the most important indicator, whereas others rely on systolic values. Generally, antihypertensive therapy would be instigated if diastolic pressure were

• **Figure 4.1** Sites
of action for the
pharmacological reduction
of blood pressure

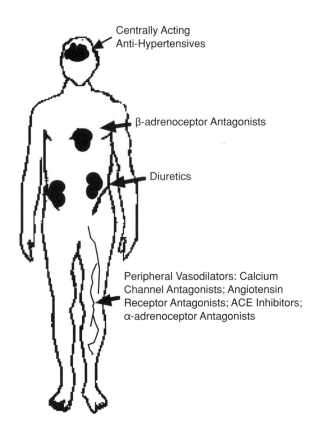

• **Figure 4.1** Sites
of action for the
pharmacological reduction
of blood pressure

Centrally Acting
Anti-Hypertensives

β-adrenoceptor Antagonists

Diuretics

Peripheral Vasodilators: Calcium
Channel Antagonists; Angiotensin
Receptor Antagonists; ACE Inhibitors;
α-adrenoceptor Antagonists

Hypertension is
symptomless

above 95 and/or systolic pressure were above 160, although some authorities recommend treatment at 140mmHg.

Drugs used to decrease blood pressure act in one or more of three basic ways: they decrease the rate and force of contractions of the heart; they decrease plasma volume or they decrease the peripheral resistance to blood flow, see figure 4.1 and Box 4.4.

■ 4.7.1 DIURETICS

Diuretic drugs act on the kidney tubule to decrease the reabsorption of sodium and therefore to promote the excretion of urine. The mechanisms of action of the various diuretic drugs is described in Chapter 5. Initiation of treatment with a diuretic results in a marked increase in urine volume and electrolyte excretion, the consequence of which is reduced extracellular fluid and plasma volumes. The ultimate effect is a reduction in cardiac output and therefore decreased blood pressure. The paradox of the treatment of hypertension with diuretic drugs, however, is that eventually the urine output and plasma volume returns to pretreatment values but the blood pressure remains decreased. Despite the uncertainty about their mechanism of action, diuretic drugs remain a first-line treatment for mild hypertension.

■ 4.7.2 β-ADRENOCEPTOR ANTAGONISTS

Antagonism of the β_1-adrenoceptor of the heart results in a reduction in the rate and force of contraction. The reduced cardiac output therefore decreases systemic blood pressure. In a manner analogous to that seen with diuretics, however, continued treatment with β-adrenoceptor antagonists such as propranolol or atenolol may be accompanied by

THE TREATMENT OF CARDIOVASCULAR DISORDERS

■ *Box 4.4* The properties of drugs commonly used for the treatment of hypertension

Action	Agent	Proprietary name
Decrease rate and force of contraction of the heart		
β-Adrenoceptor antagonists	Atenolol	Tenormin®
Decrease plasma volume		
Loop diuretic	Frusemide (furosemide)	Lasix®
Thiazide diuretic	Chlorothiazide	Saluric®
Increase circulatory volume		
ACE inhibitor	Captopril	Capoten®
Angiotensin antagonist	Losartan	Cozaar®
Nifedipine	Nifedipine	Adalat®

a return of the cardiac output to pretreatment values but a sustained reduction in blood pressure. It is therefore clear that the effects of these drugs on cardiac activity may not be the only mechanism by which they work. Another proposed mechanism of action is related to their effects on the renin–angiotensin system (see Section 4.7.3). Renin is an enzyme secreted by the juxtaglomerular apparatus of the kidney tubule in response to decreased blood supply to the kidney. The effect of renin is to initiate the production of angiotensin II, a potent vasoconstrictor. Antagonists of β-adrenoceptors reduce the secretion of renin and therefore, indirectly, reduce peripheral vasoconstriction, peripheral resistance and blood pressure. This mechanism undoubtedly contributes to the antihypertensive effects of the β-adrenoceptor antagonists, but, as evidenced by the fact that these drugs also decrease blood pressure in patients with low or normal renin concentrations, other mechanisms must also play a significant role.

A final potential mechanism of action of these drugs relates to their effects in the brain. Direct administration of β-adrenoceptor antagonists to the brain is followed by a reduction in blood pressure, indicating a central effect of these drugs. Many of this class of drugs, however, have only limited ability to penetrate the blood–brain barrier. Such drugs are still effective antihypertensives, thus indicating the non-essential nature of the central site of action for the antihypertensive effect.

In conclusion, β-adrenoceptor antagonists are widely used, effective antagonists but their mechanism of action is unclear; it is likely that all of the mechanisms described above contribute to their therapeutic actions.

■ 4.7.3 ANGIOTENSIN-CONVERTING ENZYME INHIBITORS

As described above in Section 4.7.2, the renin–angiotensin system is important in the maintenance of blood pressure, most importantly pressure within the renal artery. For many years it has been recognised that a proportion, perhaps 10%, of hypertensive patients suffered from a condition known as renal hypertension. In this condition there is a deficiency in the blood supply to the kidney which results in the secretion of renin. Renin catalyses the conversion of the inactive peptide angiotensinogen to angiotensin I, which is subsequently converted to angiotensin II by angiotensin-converting enzyme. Angiotensin II causes widespread vasoconstriction which elevates blood pressure and thus increases

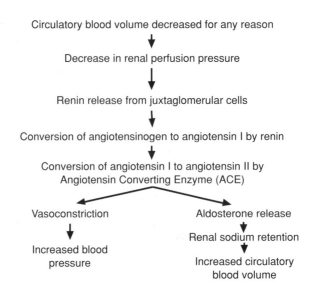

• **Figure 4.2** The renin–angiotensin system and its effect on the cardiovascular system (reproduced from Gard, P.R. (1998) *Modules in Life Science: Human Endocrinology*, London: Taylor & Francis)

Circulatory blood volume decreased for any reason

↓

Decrease in renal perfusion pressure

↓

Renin release from juxtaglomerular cells

↓

Conversion of angiotensinogen to angiotensin I by renin

↓

Conversion of angiotensin I to angiotensin II by
Angiotensin Converting Enzyme (ACE)

Vasoconstriction   Aldosterone release

↓   ↓

Increased blood   Renal sodium retention
pressure

↓

Increased circulatory
blood volume

the blood supply to the kidney (see figure 4.2). The earliest form of treatment for this form of hypertension was nephrectomy, but more recently the treatment has been the use of angiotensin-converting enzyme inhibitors (ACE inhibitors or ACEI). ACE inhibitors such as captopril and enalapril have since been shown to decrease blood pressure in the majority of hypertensive patients, particularly those with raised plasma renin. The reduction in blood pressure is a consequence of the peripheral vasodilation and the reduction in peripheral resistance; these drugs have little effect in individuals with normal blood pressure. The most noticeable adverse effect of the ACE inhibitors is the development of an irritating dry cough, which is readily reversible on withdrawal of the drug. ACE inhibitors should not be used in patients with bilateral renal stenosis (i.e. bilateral deficiency of renal blood supply) as blockade of the normal homeostatic mechanism severely reduces the blood flow to the kidney and renal failure ensues.

■ 4.7.4 ANGIOTENSIN RECEPTOR ANTAGONISTS

Angiotensin (AT$_1$) receptor antagonists such as losartan have an advantage over the ACE inhibitors in that they do not prevent the actions of angiotensin at the AT$_2$ receptor

Angiotensin (AT$_1$) receptor antagonists such as losartan intervene in the renin–angiotensin system in a manner similar to the ACE inhibitors, except that they prevent the actions of angiotensin II at its receptor rather than prevent its production. These drugs do not produce the dry cough and it has been argued that they have an advantage over the ACE inhibitors in that they do not prevent the actions of angiotensin at the AT$_2$ receptor. AT$_2$ receptors are involved with cell replication and repair, particularly in the myocardium.

■ 4.7.5 CALCIUM CHANNEL ANTAGONISTS

Calcium channel antagonists prevent the influx of calcium into smooth muscle cells, and in some cases, cardiac muscle cells; in so doing they prevent muscle contraction. Thus drugs such as dihydropyridine, which acts only on smooth muscle, reduces blood pressure by reducing peripheral resistance, whereas drugs such as verapamil and diltiazem not only reduce peripheral resistance but also decrease blood pressure by reducing cardiac output as a consequence of their effect on myocardial cells.

■ 4.7.6 OTHER PERIPHERAL VASODILATORS

There is a wide range of other drugs which decrease peripheral resistance and can be used for the treatment of hypertension. These range from the potassium ion channel openers, such as nicorandil, to the α_1-adrenoceptor antagonists, such as prazosin and indoramin. Drugs that prevent the release of noradrenaline at the sympathetic neuroeffector junction similarly prevent vasoconstriction via α_1-adrenoceptors and therefore reduce peripheral resistance. Examples of such drugs are the ganglion blocking drugs such as trimetaphan and the adrenergic neurone blocking drugs such as guanethidine. These drugs not only decrease peripheral resistance but also prevent the effects of noradrenaline on the heart, thus reducing cardiac output. Ganglion blocking drugs and adrenergic neurone blocking drugs are now rarely used because of the large number of side-effects induced by their actions at other sites of the autonomic nervous system.

As mentioned in Section 4.5, nitric oxide also acts to dilate blood vessels, although usually not to a degree sufficient to allow treatment of hypertension. Nitric oxide induces vasodilation by stimulating the synthesis of guanosine triphosphate (GTP). The anti-impotence drug sildenafil (Viagra®) inhibits phosphodiesterase, subtype 5, an enzyme responsible for the breakdown of GTP, and therefore potentiates and prolongs the effects of the nitric oxide. This subtype of phosphodiesterase is specific to the genitalia, explaining why the vasodilatory effects of sildenafil are limited to the penis with no effects on systemic blood pressure.

■ 4.7.7 CENTRALLY ACTING ANTIHYPERTENSIVE AGENTS

The final group of drugs for the treatment of hypertension are the centrally acting antihypertensive agents such as α-methyldopa and clonidine. α-Methyldopa is taken up into the noradrenergic nerve terminal where it is metabolised to α-methyl noradrenaline and released as a false transmitter; clonidine acts on presynaptic α_2-adrenoceptors to inhibit the release of noradrenaline. The net effect of these two drugs is to reduce central noradrenergic function, which results in a decrease in blood pressure. The advantage of such drugs is that they have no effect on other aspects of the autonomic system and can therefore be used in the treatment of hypertensive patients who also suffer from asthma. The disadvantage is that they disrupt the central noradrenergic system and therefore produce such side-effects as sedation and depression (see Chapter 4). These drugs are rarely used except in patients for whom the first-line treatments such as ACE inhibitors, diuretics and β-adrenoceptor antagonists have been unsuccessful, or in pregnant women in whom other classes of drugs are contraindicated.

The advantage of centrally acting antihypertensives is that they have no effect on other aspects of the autonomic system; the disadvantage is that they disrupt the central nervous system and therefore produce such side-effects as sedation and depression

■ SUMMARY

- The cardiovascular system acts to supply all tissues of the body with a constant supply of oxygen and nutrients. Any form of cardiovascular disorders results in damage to the tissue being supplied, and frequently death for the individual. Cardiovascular disease is the most common cause of death in the Western world.
- One such cardiovascular disorder is arrhythmia, in which the ordered nature of the contractions of the cardiac muscle becomes disrupted and the heart therefore fails to function as an efficient pump. Arrhythmias can be caused by damage to the conducting tissue of the heart, abnormal ionic environments and excessive cardiac stimulation. The drugs used to treat arrhythmias all act by blocking ions channels and therefore prevent the rapidly depolarising cells from depolarising or repolarising.
- The function of the heart is also compromised if its muscle is unable to contract effectively: heart failure. Many of the drugs used to treat heart failure act by either preventing the pacemaker cells from maintaining their depolarised state or by mimicking or enhancing

the actions of natural transmitters which stimulate the heart. The deleterious effects of heart failure can also be reduced by decreasing the work-load of the heart, for example by use of peripheral vasodilators or diuretics.

■ Peripheral vasodilators are also used to decrease the work-load of the heart and to increase the flow of blood through the coronary blood vessels in the relief of angina.

■ The most common cardiovascular disorder is hypertension. This condition is symptomless but is known to be related to later conditions such as thrombosis, stroke and kidney failure, which are often fatal. Drugs used in the treatment of hypertension act via a variety of mechanisms. Diuretic drugs act to increase the excretion of ions and water and therefore decrease the plasma volume and, as a consequence, cardiac output; β-adrenoceptor antagonists act directly on the heart to decrease cardiac output. The majority of other antihypertensive drugs decrease blood pressure by reducing peripheral resistance, either by blocking the production or actions of angiotensin II, by blocking calcium channels or by disrupting the actions of the sympathetic nervous system.

■ REVISION QUESTIONS

For each question select the most appropriate answer. Correct answers are presented in Appendix 1.

1. Which of the following is *not* a mechanism of action of an antiarrhythmic drug:
    (a) sodium ion channel blockade;
    (b) calcium ion channel blockade;
    (c) potassium ion channel blockade;
    (d) chloride ion channel blockade;
    (e) β-adrenoceptor antagonism.

2. Cardiac glycosides relieve heart failure by:
    (a) inhibition of Na^+,K^+-ATPase;
    (b) reduction of peripheral vascular resistance;
    (c) potassium ion channel blockade;
    (d) chloride ion channel blockade;
    (e) stimulation of β-adrenoceptors.

3. In the relief of angina, glyceryl trinitrate acts by:
    (a) blocking calcium ion channels;
    (b) stimulating the synthesis of cAMP;
    (c) increasing nitric oxide concentrations;
    (d) β-adrenoceptor antagonism;
    (e) inhibition of Na^+,K^+-ATPase.

4. Angiotensin-converting enzyme inhibitors reduce blood pressure by:
    (a) preventing the effects of angiotensin II on the heart;
    (b) blocking the effects of angiotensin II on peripheral blood vessels;
    (c) preventing the metabolism of angiotensin II;
    (d) preventing the synthesis of angiotensin II;
    (e) preventing the release of renin.

5. Which of the following could *not* be used in the treatment of hypertension:
    (a) $β_2$-adrenoceptor antagonists;
    (b) $α_1$-adrenoceptor antagonists;

(c)   angiotensin receptor antagonists;

(d)   calcium channel antagonists;

(e) β_1-adrenoceptor antagonists.

6.   Which of the following would be expected to elevate blood pressure:

(a) β_2-adrenoceptor agonists;

(b) β_1-adrenoceptor antagonists;

(c) α_1-adrenoceptor agonists;

(d) α_2-adrenoceptor antagonists;

(e) α_1-adrenoceptor antagonists.

■ SELECTED READING

Akera, Tai and Brody, T.M. (1998) Drugs to treat heart failure: cardiac glycosides. In Brody, T.M., Larner, J. and Minneman, K.P. (eds) *Human Pharmacology: Molecular to Clinical* (Third edition), (St. Louis: Mosby), 213–226.

Fink, G.D. (1998) Antihypertensive drugs. In Brody, T.M., Larner, J. and Minneman, K.P. (eds) *Human Pharmacology: Molecular to Clinical* (Third edition), (St. Louis: Mosby), 181–194.

Galbraith, A., Bullock, S., Manias, E., Hunt, B. and Richards, A. (1999) Digitalis, antiarrhythmic and anti-anginal drugs. In Galbraith, A., Bullock, S., Manias, E., Hunt, B. and Richards, A. *Fundamentals of Pharmacology*, (Harlow: Addison Wesley Longman), 369–385.

Galbraith, A., Bullock, S., Manias, E., Hunt, B. and Richards, A. (1999) Antihypertensive drugs. In Galbraith, A., Bullock, S., Manias, E., Hunt, B. and Richards, A. *Fundamentals of Pharmacology*, (Harlow: Addison Wesley Longman), 386–398.

Hume, J.R and Woosley, R.L. (1998) Cardiac electrophysiology and antiarrhythmic agents. In Brody, T. M., Larner, J. and Minneman, K.P. (eds) *Human Pharmacology: Molecular to Clinical* (Third edition), (St. Louis: Mosby), 195–212.

Martini, F.H. (1998) The heart. In Martini, F.H. *Fundamentals of Anatomy and Physiology* (Fourth edition), (New Jersey: Prentice Hall), 672–707.

Martini, F.H. (1998) Blood vessels and circulation. In Martini, F.H. *Fundamentals of Anatomy and Physiology* (Fourth edition), (New Jersey: Prentice Hall), 708–768.

Rang, H.P., Dale, M.M. and Ritter, J.M. (1999) The heart. In Rang, H.P., Dale, M.M. and Ritter, J.M. *Pharmacology* (Fourth edition), (Edinburgh: Churchill Livingstone), 250–277.

Rang, H.P., Dale, M.M. and Ritter, J.M. (1999) The vascular system. In Rang, H.P., Dale, M.M. and Ritter, J.M. *Pharmacology* (Fourth edition), (Edinburgh: Churchill Livingstone), 278–300.

Vaghy, P.L. (1998) Calcium antagonists. In Brody, T.M., Larner, J. and Minneman, K.P. (eds) *Human Pharmacology: Molecular to Clinical* (Third edition), (St. Louis: Mosby), 227–238.

Westfall, D.P., Gerthoffer, W.T. and Webb, R.C. (1998) Vasodilators and nitric oxide. In Brody, T.M., Larner, J. and Minneman, K.P. (eds) *Human Pharmacology: Molecular to Clinical* (Third edition), (St. Louis: Mosby), 239–248.

■ COMPUTER-AIDED LEARNING PACKAGES

Further details of these learning packages can be found at
http://www.coacs.com/PCCAL/

CardiovascularSystem/Autonomic Nervous System Tutor (version 3.0), Pharmacy Consortium for Computer Aided Learning (PCCAL), COACS Ltd, University of Bath.

Hypertension (version 2.0), Pharmacy Consortium for Computer Aided Learning (PCCAL), COACS Ltd, University of Bath.

DRUGS AFFECTING THE BLOOD AND ITS COMPOSITION

■ 5.1 INTRODUCTION

The blood is comprised of the aqueous plasma component and the cellular components. Plasma is an aqueous solution that acts to transport water-soluble chemicals (hormones, nutrients, etc.) around the body. In many cases, however, the chemicals that require transport are lipids, or lipid soluble; in these cases the substances are rendered more water soluble by binding to plasma proteins. Plasma proteins also play an important role in maintaining the osmolarity of the blood, thus ensuring that fluid does not move into the tissues by osmosis, and in haemostasis. Haemostasis is the process by which blood is maintained within the blood vessels, in a fluid state. The best-known aspect of haemostasis is blood clotting, but there are other aspects.

The cellular components of blood are the red blood cells, or erythrocytes, the white blood cells, or leukocytes, and the platelets. The primary function of erythrocytes is transport of oxygen which binds to haemoglobin contained within them. Leukocytes are involved in defence mechanisms, such as antibody formation, and the platelets are important in haemostasis.

There are several groups of drugs that can alter the activity and composition of the blood. These range from drugs that act on the kidney to influence the fluid and ionic composition of the plasma, through drugs that influence the lipid components of the plasma, to drugs that have effects on the production, composition and activity of the cellular components of the blood. Each of these classes of drug will be discussed in turn.

Any disruption of bone marrow activity, for example following administration of cytotoxic drugs, has the effect of interfering with blood cell formation

■ 5.2 DRUGS ACTING ON BLOOD CELL FORMATION AND ACTIVITY

Erythrocytes, leukocytes and platelets are all derived from bone marrow, although each cell subtype is derived from bone marrow at different sites of the body; certain types of leukocyte are also derived from lymphoid tissues such as the thymus gland. Any disruption of bone marrow activity, for example following administration of cytotoxic drugs, has the effect of interfering with blood cell formation and therefore has a profound effect on the function of the whole body. Disorders of blood cell formation and the drugs used for their treatment are discussed below.

■ *Box 5.1* Some possible causes of anaemia

Thalassaemia

Ionising radiation

Iron-deficient diet

Folic acid deficiency

Vitamin B_{12} deficiency

Erythropoietin deficiency (e.g. renal disease)

Haemorrhage (e.g. trauma, menstruation, gastric ulcer)

Deficient iron absorption (e.g. gastrointestinal disorder)

Depression of bone marrow (e.g. due to anticancer drugs)

Haemolysis (e.g. adverse drug reaction or immune response)

■ 5.2.1 ERYTHROCYTES

The formation of erythrocytes (erythropoiesis) is one of the most active processes in adults: approximately two hundred billion (2×10^{11}) new erythrocytes are formed each day. Erthrocytes are formed in bone marrow, although in the fetus, before the bones are formed, the erythrocytes are formed by the blood vessels themselves and by the liver, kidney, spleen and muscles. In children, the bone marrow of all bones is involved in erythrocyte production, but in adults only the bones of the trunk, for example pelvis, sternum and skull, retain that function.

The active life span of an erythrocyte is 120 days, so there is a complete 'turn-over' of erythrocytes every 4 months. Aged erythrocytes are removed by the reticulo-endothelial system, predominantly in the spleen.

The normal erythrocyte concentration is approximately 5 thousand billion cells per litre of blood, and this remains fairly constant. It is therefore clear that the rate of erythrocyte formation matches the rate of degradation, although there are sometimes increases or decreases in erythrocyte concentrations under certain circumstances. The stimulus for erythropoiesis is oxygen deficiency, hypoxia, which can occur in conditions such as lung disease or at high altitude. Within a few hours of the onset of hypoxia a glycoprotein hormone called erythropoietin is secreted by juxtatubular cells of the kidney. Erythropoietin causes the production of more erythrocytes from the bone marrow.

One special form of oxygen deficiency is anaemia. Anaemia refers to a condition in which there is a reduced concentration of haemoglobin in the blood. Haemoglobin is the iron-containing molecule that is present in erythrocytes and which is responsible for the transport of oxygen. A deficiency of haemoglobin results in an inability to transport oxygen, which is therefore analogous to a situation of hypoxia. All forms of anaemia, except that associated with kidney failure, are accompanied by an increase in the secretion of erythropoietin. Anaemia can take several forms and has several causes (Box 5.1). The most common form of anaemia is the iron-deficiency anaemia that is caused by blood loss such as menstruation or childbirth.

Iron deficiency initially causes a deficiency in the synthesis of haemoglobin, resulting in a decrease in the mean haemoglobin content of the erythrocytes. Prolonged iron deficiency causes a decrease in the number of erythrocytes. The body normally contains about 3–4g of iron, of which about 70% is contained within haemoglobin, most of the remaining iron is in storage. About 1mg of iron is lost per day in urine, faeces or desquamated cells in males and females, but in females there is an additional loss of about 25mg of

Anaemia is any condition in which there is a reduced concentration of haemoglobin in the blood iron per month with the blood loss of menstruation. A normal female therefore loses an average of approximately 2mg of iron per day. Additional factors that deplete iron are pregnancy (700mg over 9 months), breast feeding (0.5mg per day) or any form of haemorrhage. There are no mechanisms for the control of iron loss, therefore the only way in which the body can maintain an iron balance is to control iron absorption. The average dietary intake of iron is 14mg per day, of which only 10% is absorbed.

Much of the dietary iron is absorbed in the form of haem from meat. Having been absorbed from the gut contents, the iron becomes bound either to apoferritin to form ferritin, a storage form of iron which remains within the mucosal cell and may eventually be lost by desquamation, or to transferrin which transports the iron to the bone marrow. It is because of the relatively greater binding of iron to apoferritin than to transferrin that only about 10% of dietary iron is absorbed; at times of reduced iron intake the synthesis of apoferritin decreases, resulting in an increased percentage uptake of iron.

Most forms of iron-deficiency anaemia can be treated by administration of oral iron such as ferrous sulphate or ferrous gluconate

Most forms of iron-deficiency anaemia can be treated by administration of oral iron. The iron is given in the form of a salt such as ferrous sulphate or ferrous gluconate, but there are minor differences in the absorption of the different salts. In individuals where the iron deficiency is a result of a malabsorption condition or due to bowel disease the iron is given by injection.

Hyperchromic anaemia may also occur if there is an abnormality in haemoglobin synthesis, rather than iron incorporation. Some forms of haemoglobinopathies respond to treatment with vitamin B_6 (pyridoxine).

The other forms of anaemia are the megaloblastic anaemias. Megaloblastic anaemia is a condition in which the erythrocytes fail to develop correctly, resulting in over-sized, dysfunctional cells. Megaloblastic anaemias are caused by a deficiency of either folic acid or vitamin B_{12} (cobalamins). Folic acid is essential for the synthesis of DNA and B_{12} is important for cell maturation and for the promotion of folic acid uptake by the bone marrow. Deficiency of B_{12} affects production of all cells and therefore affects not only the blood but also other systems, such as the nervous system.

One early treatment for megaloblastic anaemia was to eat raw liver

An important feature of vitamin B_{12} is that it is abundant in the normal diet, but it requires a chemical called intrinsic factor of Castle for it to be absorbed. This intrinsic factor is normally present in the stomach. One early treatment for megaloblastic anaemia was to eat raw liver. It was later found that the efficacy of this therapy was a consequence of liver containing not only B_{12} but also folic acid and intrinsic factor of Castle. A more recent therapy is the administration of B_{12}, either with or without folic acid, but by injection, thus avoiding the requirement for the intrinsic factor.

Anaemia may also be a consequence of kidney damage, because of the failure to secrete erythropoietin. In such cases the patients can be treated with epoetin (NeoRecormon®), which is a version of human erythropoietin produced by recombinant technology.

■ 5.2.2 LEUKOCYTES

Leukocytes are divided into several subtypes: approximately 70% of the leukocytes are granulocytes. Granulocytes are further subdivided into neutrophils (95%), eosinophils (4%) and basophils (1%). When basophils leave the blood vessels and enter the tissues they are known as mast cells. All of these cells are involved in the body's defence mechanisms; for example, neutrophils are phagocytic. The remaining leukocytes are lymphocytes, which are important in antibody production, and monocytes, which again are phagocytic. All leukocytes are formed from bone marrow although lymphocytes are also produced by lymphoid tissues such as the thymus gland.

White blood cell counts may be raised within hours of violent exercise, fever or haem-orrhage, this production of leukocytes may be due to colony stimulating factors, such as granulocyte-colony-stimulating factor which is produced by monocytes. Therapeutic-ally, these factors can be admministered to potentiate leukocyte production in order to overcome the effects of some anticancer drugs which normally decrease white blood cell counts. Examples of colony-stimulating factors are filgrastim (Neupogen®), lenograstim (Granocyte®) and molgramostim (Leucomax®).

■ 5.3 DRUGS AFFECTING HAEMOSTASIS

Haemostasis is the process by which blood is kept within the blood vessels in a fluid state. Any damage to a blood vessel can result in leakage of blood, this leaked blood invariably coagulates, thus temporarily sealing the damaged blood vessel and limiting the extent of blood loss. Blood can, however, sometimes coagulate inappropriately, which results in blockage of the blood vessel and deprivation of the tissues of oxygen and nutrients. In order to limit the extent of damage caused by inappropriate blood coagulation, the body is able to break down the clot (fibrinolysis); there is therefore a constant, ongoing pro-cess of coagulation and fibrinolysis.

The immediate consequence of damage to a blood vessel is vasoconstriction, this is then followed by platelet activation and adhesion to form a haemostatic plug, this plug is then usually strengthened and replaced by fibrin. If the process occurs in a blood vessel that is not leaking, it is termed thrombosis. Factors that may precipitate thrombosis are changes to the blood vessel wall, for example atheromatous plaques, or changes to the blood flow, for example turbulence or stasis. The characteristics of the thrombi depend on the site of their formation: arterial thrombi are composed of platelets and leukocytes entrapped in a fibrin mesh, whereas venous thrombi are composed of erythrocytes within the fibrin web. If an artery or arteriole becomes blocked by a thrombus, the tissue that it normally supplies becomes ischaemic and may die, an example of this is myocardial infarction, where a coronary artery becomes blocked, resulting in damage to the cardiac tissue. An embolus is a fragment of a thrombus that breaks free and travels with the blood flow until it blocks a narrow vessel.

Platelet activation occurs following tissue damage or inflammation. Activated plate-lets aggregate and adhere to form platelet plugs; they also change shape from a smooth disc to a spiky sphere and they release mediators such as 5-HT, ADP and some coagula-tion factors (see later). Inappropriate formation of the platelet plug due to the presence of atherosclerosis is a major cause of thrombosis. Changes in the blood vessel walls, and activation of platelets, are also responsible for the activation of the blood clotting cascade.

Blood clots are formed from fibrin, which is an insoluble, long-chain protein; it is normally present in plasma in the form of fibrinogen, a soluble protein. The conversion of fibrinogen to fibrin is brought about by the enzyme thrombin. Fibrin is further stab-ilised by the presence of fibrin stabilising factor, or factor XIII. Thrombin is normally present in the form of the inactive prothrombin; the conversion of prothrombin to thrombin requires the presence of calcium and thromboplastin (also called thrombokinase or activ-ated factor X). Activation of factor X is the culmination of a complex cascade process involving several other clotting factors. This cascade process is initiated either by changes in the characteristics of the blood vessel wall (called the intrinsic system) or by tissue damage or activation of platelets (the extrinsic system). The coagulation cascade is pre-sented in figure 5.1; it should be remembered that each stage of the cascade results in an amplification of the process, thus a single stimulus may result in the synthesis of many millions of fibrin molecules.

Haemostasis is the process by which blood is kept within the blood vessels in a fluid state

Inappropriate formation of the platelet plug due to the presence of atherosclerosis is a major cause of thrombosis

• **Figure 5.1** The cascade process responsible for blood clotting

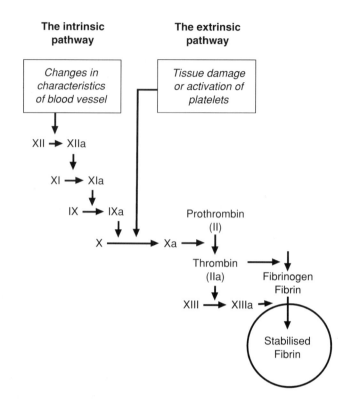

The intrinsic pathway

The extrinsic pathway

Changes in characteristics of blood vessel

Tissue damage or activation of platelets

XII → XIIa

XI → XIa

IX → IXa

Prothrombin (II)

X ——→ Xa →

Thrombin (IIa) ——→

Fibrinogen
Fibrin

XIII → XIIIa →

Stabilised Fibrin

Haemophilia is a group of conditions in which there is an inherited deficiency of one (or more) of the coagulation factors. Vitamin K deficiency may also precipitate disorders of coagulation, due to its requirement for the synthesis of many of the clotting factors. Inherited haemophilia is treated by infusion of fresh plasma containing the required factors, or by administration of more concentrated solutions of those factors.

■ 5.3.1 ANTIPLATELET DRUGS

There is good evidence to indicate that the incidence of arterial thrombosis can be decreased by prevention of inappropriate platelet activation. Aspirin irreversibly inhibits cyclo-oxygenase (COX-1, see Chapter 9), and therefore inhibits the synthesis of thromboxane-A_2 by platelets and prostacyclin by the endothelium. Because the endothelium is able to synthesis more cyclo-oxygenase, unlike the platelets, the overall effect is to alter the ratio of thromboxane-A_2 to prostacyclin, which reduces platelet aggregation. The effect of the single dose of aspirin lasts for the life span of the platelet (7–10 days) and therefore aspirin therapy need only be intermittent. Low-dose aspirin, administered daily, is now a recognised therapy for the prevention of platelet aggregation and thus prevention of thrombotic cerebrovascular or cardiovascular disease.

Low-dose aspirin, administered daily, is now a recognised therapy for the prevention of platelet aggregation and thus prevention of thrombotic cerebrovascular or cardiovascular disease

Other antiplatelet drugs, which act by preventing a variety of platelet-activating stimuli, include dipyridamole (Persantin®) and clopidogrel (Plavix®).

■ 5.3.2 ANTICOAGULANT AGENTS

Venous thrombosis is treated or prevented by use of the anticoagulant agents. These agents are also used prophylactically to prevent thrombus formation following insertion of a medical device such as an artificial heart valve or replacement hip. There are two classes of anticoagulant drugs, the oral anticoagulants and the injectable agents.

The oral anticoagulants reduce the effects of vitamin K; this vitamin is required for the synthesis of several of the clotting factors, for example factors II, VII, IX and X. Because of this mechanism of action, these agents are not effective *in vitro*, and their effects take several days to develop, dependent on the natural turnover of the relevant clotting factors. The most important member of this group of drugs is warfarin, although the related compounds nicoumalone (Sinthrome®) and phenindione (Dindevan®) are also available. The major risk of anticoagulant therapy is the risk of thrombus formation if the dose is insufficient or bleeding if the dose is excessive. Anticoagulant therapy therefore requires careful monitoring of the dose and response, an exercise made more difficult by the fact that warfarin is metabolised by liver enzymes that may be induced by drugs such as carbamazepine (Chapter 3) and inhibited by drugs such as cimetidine (Chapter 7).

The injectable anticoagulants such as heparin act by activating antithrombin III, an endogenous factor that inhibits the actions of thrombin, factor X and factors IX, XI and XII. Heparin itself is a collection of related chemicals with molecular weights ranging from 4000 to 40,000. These different heparins have differential effects on the various clotting factors, but are all equally therapeutically useful. Because of their chemical structure, the heparins are not orally active and therefore have to be given by injection, the low molecular weight heparins have a longer duration of action than standard (mixed) heparin. As with the oral anticoagulants, the major difficulty of treatment with the heparins is the titration of dose against effect, although an additional problem is the possibility of antiheparin antibody formation at the site of injection; heparin can also induce thrombocytopenia (platelet deficiency).

A newer injectable anticoagulant is lepirudin (Refludan®) which is based upon the anticoagulant secreted by the leech. Lepirudin is a direct inhibitor of thrombin and is used in patients with heparin-induced thrombocytopenia who require anticoagulant therapy.

■ 5.3.3 FIBRINOLYTIC AGENTS

Once the fibrin of a clot or thrombus has formed, it must eventually be removed, for example for replacement by connective tissue. The liquefaction of the clot is called fibrinolysis and it may occur as rapidly as the initial coagulation. The enzyme responsible for removal of the fibrin is plasmin, which also degrades several of the clotting factors. The precursor of plasmin is plasminogen and its conversion to plasmin is stimulated by plasminogen activators which are produced as part of the haemostatic process to limit the extent of the coagulation.

Fibrinolytic drugs (Box 5.2) act to stimulate plasmin and are used to remove thrombi or emboli and therefore to re-open occluded blood vessels. There is now very good evidence that prompt administration of one of these 'clot busters' significantly increases the survival rate following thrombotic cerebrovascular or cardiovascular events.

■ 5.3.4 ANTIFIBRINOLYTIC AGENTS

There are a small number of clinical situations in which it is desirable to prevent the normal breakdown of the fibrin plug and therefore to extend the effective 'life span' of the fibrin plug and to limit blood loss. The most common of such conditions are menorrhagia (excessive menstrual blood loss) and following tooth extraction. Tranexamic acid (Cyklokapron®) inhibits plasminogen activation and therefore prevents clot removal and aprotinin (Trasylol®) is a protease inhibitor which prevents the inactivation of plasmin. Ethamsylate (etamsylate; Dicynene®) acts by limiting capillary leakage of blood, although the mechanism of action is unknown.

■ *Box 5.2* Fibrinolytic drugs used for the removal of blood clots

Agent	*Proprietary name*
Alteplase	Actilyse®
Anistreplase	Eminase®
Reteplase	Rapilysin®
Streptokinase	Kabikinase®
	Streptase®

■ 5.4 DRUGS AFFECTING PLASMA COMPOSITION

The ionic composition of the urine is controlled predominantly by the kidney, which regulates both the reabsorption of water and of ions such as sodium, potassium and calcium. The kidney is also responsible for regulation of blood pH. The carbohydrate composition of the plasma is regulated by pancreatic hormones, hepatic enzyme activity and digestive processes and metabolic enzyme activity.

■ 5.4.1 DIURETIC AND ANTIDIURETIC DRUGS

Before it is possible to appreciate the mechanisms of action of the various diuretic drugs, it is first necessary to understand the processes by which the kidney regulates the ionic composition of the plasma. Detailed coverage of this subject matter is beyond the scope of this text, but the various processes will be described in summary. The more interested reader should consult a textbook of physiology.

The kidney is comprised of millions of nephrons or tubules, each of which acts to filter the plasma and to reabsorb selectively 'valuable' solutes; solutes that are not reabsorbed are excreted in the urine. The structure of the nephron is presented in figure 5.2. Initially, plasma is filtered at the glomerulus, where all of the components of the blood other than the blood cells and the large plasma proteins enter the tubule; approximately 180 litres of filtrate are produced per day. The next process that occurs is within the proximal tubule, where there is active reabsorption of many of the solutes back into the blood vessel; approximately 90% of the sodium, chloride and water content of the tubule is reabsorbed at this point, with all of the glucose and amino acids being reabsorbed. There are no uptake processes for urea, thus this waste product remains within the tubule for later disposal. The proximal tubule is also the site for tubular secretion; this is where moieties that are normally bound to plasma proteins, and therefore not filtered at the glomerulus, are stripped from the proteins and secreted into the tubule. One example of such a moiety is penicillin. By the time the tubular fluid leaves the proximal tubule to enter the loop of Henle there has been little change in composition other than a decrease in glucose and amino acid concentration and an increase in urea concentration, but the volume has decreased by about 90%.

The next portion of the kidney tubule is the loop of Henle, this structure possesses a $Na^+, K^+, 2Cl^-$ ion co-transport system, which causes the removal of Na^+ and Cl^- from the tubule into the blood; water is prevented from following the ions passively by the nature of the tubule walls at this site. The loop of Henle does not play a role in regulating the ionic balance of the plasma, but it is essential for the process of water reabsorption (see later).

After the loop of Henle the tubular fluid enters the distal tubule, at which site the sodium ions are reabsorbed in exchange for potassium. This sodium reabsorption is under

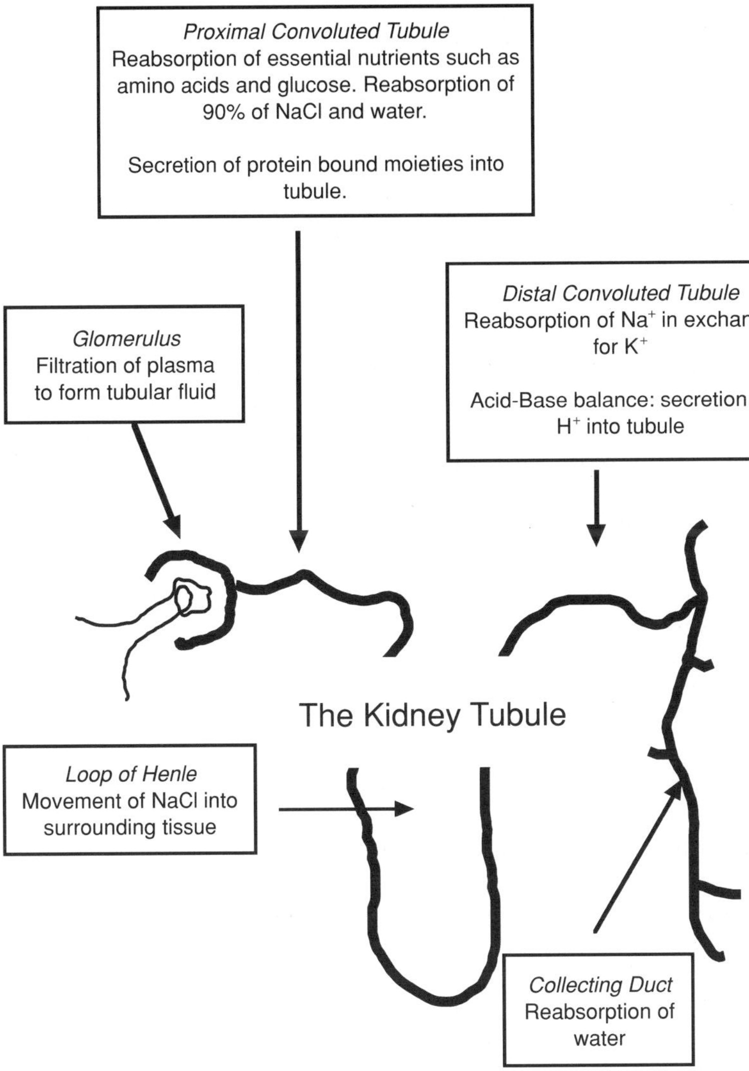

• **Figure 5.2** The role of the nephron in the formation of urine

Proximal Convoluted Tubule
Reabsorption of essential nutrients such as amino acids and glucose. Reabsorption of 90% of NaCl and water.

Secretion of protein bound moieties into tubule.

Distal Convoluted Tubule
Reabsorption of Na^+ in exchange for K^+

Acid-Base balance: secretion of H^+ into tubule

Glomerulus
Filtration of plasma to form tubular fluid

The Kidney Tubule

Loop of Henle
Movement of NaCl into surrounding tissue

Collecting Duct
Reabsorption of water

the control of aldosterone. Calcium reabsorption also occurs at the distal tubule, under the control of parathyroid hormone. The distal tubule is also the site of 'acidification' of the urine, as H^+ ions are secreted into the tubule in exchange for Na^+ ions.

The final process occurs in the collecting duct; it is here that the reabsorption of water is controlled. Because of the activity of the loop of Henle, the blood vessels surrounding the collecting duct have high concentrations of Na^+ and Cl^-. Therefore there is an osmotic gradient that enables the reabsorption of water from the collecting duct into the blood vessels. This process, however, is limited by the permeability of the collecting-duct walls. In the absence of antidiuretic hormone, the walls have very low permeability to water, and therefore most of the water is excreted. Antidiuretic hormone acts to increase the permeability of the collecting duct walls and therefore to promote water reabsorption; this has the effect of decreasing the volume of urine excreted. The normal daily volume of urine is approximately 1 litre.

A diuretic drug may be defined as any compound that causes the excretion of an increased volume of urine

A diuretic drug may be defined as any compound that causes the excretion of an increased volume of urine; although a more precise definition would be a drug that increases the excretion of both fluid and solutes. Diuretics are used therapeutically in the treatment of a variety of conditions, for example hypertension, oedema and heart failure. They may also be used simply to increase the volume of urine, for example to prevent the accumulation of toxic drugs within the bladder.

Possibly the most simple of the diuretics is water. As the intake of water is increased, under normal conditions, the excretion of water increases. The process is controlled by antidiuretic hormone (ADH) from the posterior pituitary gland. ADH is secreted at times when the ionic concentration (osmolarity) of the plasma is increased, it acts on the collecting ducts of the nephron to increase the reabsorption of water, therefore decreasing the osmolarity of the plasma and decreasing the volume of urine. If there is excessive fluid intake, the osmolarity of the plasma is decreased, resulting in inhibition of the secretion of ADH and therefore causing an increase in urine volume. In diabetes insipidus there is a deficiency of ADH which causes the excretion of large volumes of urine. This condition can be treated by the administration of ADH (Chapter 8).

Unlike water, true diuretic drugs increase the excretion of both solutes and fluid. There are five major classes of diuretic agents: osmotic diuretics, carbonic anhydrase inhibitors, loop diuretics, thiazides and aldosterone antagonists; each of these groups will be covered separately. The sites of action of the various classes of diuretic drug are presented in figure 5.3.

5.4.1.1 Osmotic diuretics

Osmotic diuretics are metabolically inert substances, but they possess the important property of being filtered at the glomerulus and of not being reabsorbed from the nephron. Following administration, which is usually by intravenous injection, the substance is not utilised at all by the body and is simply excreted unchanged in the urine. Its presence in the urine exerts an osmotic pressure and therefore causes an increase in the volume of the urine. Excretion of these substances is therefore accompanied by excretion of an increased volume of fluid.

The major adverse effect of osmotic diuretics is that their presence in the blood also exerts an osmotic pressure and therefore increases the plasma volume, such an action is contraindicated in conditions such as hypertension. The only osmotic diuretic currently used therapeutically is mannitol, which is used to decrease cerebral oedema.

5.4.1.2 Carbonic anhydrase inhibitors

The enzyme carbonic anhydrase is found in high concentrations in the cells of the proximal tubule of the nephron, where it normally catalyses the ionisation of carbonic acid to H^+ and HCO_3^-. The H^+ is then transported into the tubular lumen in exchange for sodium ions. Inhibition of carbonic anhydrase reduces the availability of H^+ and therefore reduces Na^+ reabsorption. The ultimate effect of the carbonic anhydrase inhibitors, for example acetazolamide, is to increase the excretion of sodium ions, normally in combination with bicarbonate ions, and therefore to increase the excretion of fluid by osmosis. These drugs are only weakly diuretic, and are therefore rarely used as such, but they also cause excretion of HCO_3^-, which may be of use in the treatment of alkalosis.

5.4.1.3 Loop diuretics

Loop diuretics are the most potent diuretics used, hence they are sometimes known as 'high-ceiling' diuretics. These drugs act to inhibit the $Na^+, K^+, 2Cl^-$ co-transporter, which

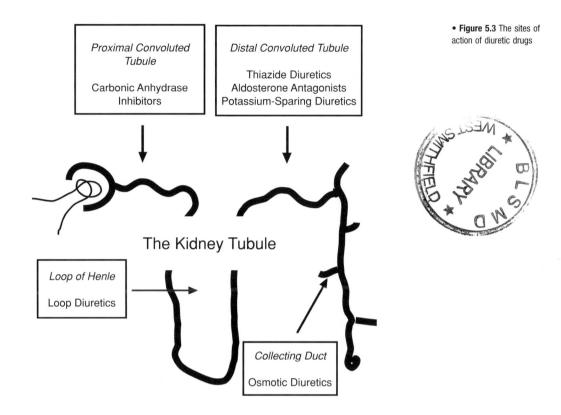

• **Figure 5.3** The sites of action of diuretic drugs

results in the retention of sodium and chloride within the tubule. The effects of this are twofold: first, there is more sodium within the tubule which, when excreted, takes with it water by osmosis; secondly, there is less sodium and chloride within the blood vessels that surround the collecting duct, thus there is less osmotic potential for the reabsorption of water at that site. These drugs produce a profound and rapid diuresis which onsets about 1 hour after oral administration and lasts for about 4 hours. In a normal person, a single dose of a loop diuretic can increase the volume of urine from 200ml to 1200ml over 3 hours.

In a normal person a single dose of a loop diuretic can increase the volume of urine from 200ml to 1200ml over 3 hours

Most of the adverse effects of the clinically used loop diuretics (Box 5.3) are related to their diuretic effects; for example, they may cause dehydration if the patient does not have sufficient fluid replacement. Another feature of these drugs is that they may cause potassium depletion. The reason for this is that they increase the amount of sodium that enters the distal tubule from the loop of Henle, this sodium is then 'exchanged' for potassium, which is excreted. This hypokalaemia may be prevented by co-administration of potassium supplements. Fortunately, there are few problems of long-term toxicity of loop diuretics because they induce their own excretion: loop diuretics are transported bound to proteins in the plasma, they are secreted into the proximal tubule and excreted in the urine. Their effect of increasing urinary output therefore increases their own excretion.

5.4.1.4 Thiazides

The thiazide diuretics (Box 5.3) act in the distal tubule to inhibit the Na^+,Cl^- co-transporter, the result of which is to increase the concentration of sodium within the tubule. These drugs have no effect on the Na^+,K^+ exchange process, so that some of the

■ *Box 5.3* Common loop and thiazide diuretics

Agent	*Proprietary name*
Loop diuretics	
Frusemide	Lasix®
(furosemide)	
Bumetanide	Burinex®
Ethacrynic acid	Edecrin®
(etacrynic acid)	
Torasemide	Torem®
Thiazide diuretics	
Chlorthiazide	Saluric®
(chlorothiazide)	
Chlortalidone	Hygroton®
Cyclopenthiazide	Navidrex®
Hydrochlorthiazide	HydroSaluric®
(hydrochlorothiazide)	
Mefruside	Baycaron®
Metolazone	Metenix®
Polythiazide	Nephril®
Xipamide	Diurexan®

extra sodium is exchanged for potassium, resulting in increased excretion of sodium, potassium and chloride ions. The presence of these extra ions within the collecting duct decreases the osmotic gradient between the tubule and the blood, and therefore reduces the ability to reabsorb water.

Thiazide diuretics also cause vasodilation, which is itself beneficial in the treatment of hypertension and may also explain the paradoxical effect of thiazides in reducing urine output in diabetes insipidus, possibly due to a decreased glomerular filtration rate.

These drugs are moderately effective diuretics with a long duration of action (up to 24 hours). Their predominant adverse effect is that of hypokalaemia, which may be prevented by co-administration of potassium supplements.

5.4.1.5 Aldosterone antagonists and potassium-sparing diuretics

As the name suggests, these agents are competitive antagonists of aldosterone, thus they prevent the ability of that hormone to promote reabsorption of sodium in exchange for potassium. The diuretic effect is due to the increased concentrations of sodium in the tubular fluid, although the effect may take several days to develop. These drugs are only used for the treatment of primary hyperaldosteronism and some forms of oedema; they are not used for the treatment of hypertension because of fears that they may increase the incidence of cancer, although this effect has only been observed in rats. Paradoxically, unlike the other diuretics, because of the mechanisms of action of aldosterone antagonists, another adverse effect is the possibility of hyperkalaemia. The archetypal aldosterone antagonist is spironolactone, although this is metabolised to a more active moiety, canrenoate, which is also available.

Triamterene and amiloride are weak diuretics which also act to prevent sodium reabsorption in exchange for potassium, probably at the ion channel normally controlled by aldosterone. These agents are of little therapeutic use alone, but they are useful in combination with other potassium-depleting diuretics as they limit the degree of hypokalaemia.

5.4.1.6 Drugs affecting antidiuretic hormone

As described above, antidiuretic hormone (ADH) controls the reabsorption of water from the collecting duct. A deficiency of ADH, or a lack of response to ADH, results in a condition called diabetes insipidus, in which there is excessive excretion of urine. If the disorder is due to a deficiency of ADH, the condition is treated by administration of ADH. If the condition is due to failure of the kidney to respond to ADH, the urinary volume can be decreased by use of a thiazide diuretic (see above). It should also be noted that alcohol has the ability to suppress ADH secretion, and therefore has a marked, reversible, diuretic effect. Nicotine potentiates ADH secretion and therefore reduces urine volume.

Alcohol has the ability to suppress ADH secretion; nicotine potentiates ADH secretion

■ 5.4.2 LIPID-LOWERING AGENTS

The total body content of cholesterol is about 125g, of which 90% is present as components of the cell membrane. This cholesterol is obtained either from the diet or from *de novo* synthesis, usually in the adrenal glands or in the liver. Dietary cholesterol is absorbed from the gut and transported to the liver, where much of it is converted to bile salts which are then secreted back into the gut. These bile salts are important for the emulsification of dietary lipids and cholesterol prior to absorption, and indeed reabsorption of the bile salts themselves accounts for a large proportion of the cholesterol intake. Cholesterol and other lipids are transported within the blood as lipoprotein particles; these have a lipid core with a protein shell. There are several types of lipoprotein particle, ranging from chylomicrons, which are the largest, to the high-density lipoproteins (HDLs), which are the smallest.

Chylomicrons are formed within the gut wall and are the major means by which dietary cholesterol is absorbed and transported to adipose tissue. The triglycerides and fatty acids are then released from the chylomicron by the actions of lipoprotein lipase; the remnants of the chylomicron are then taken up into the liver. The cholesterol that is synthesised *de novo* is initially transported in the form of very low-density lipoproteins (VLDLs), which are smaller than the chylomicrons. Again, the components of the VLDLs are liberated by the actions of lipoprotein lipase but, in this case, the remnants of the VLDL become a low-density lipoprotein (LDL) which is much smaller than the VLDL. LDLs combine with specific receptors on cell membranes which result in the LDL being transported into the cell. The receptors are then recycled and the LDL is broken down to liberate free cholesterol. The final form of lipoproteins are the high-density lipoproteins (HDLs), which are formed either in the liver or as part of the process of the lipolysis of chylomicrons or VLDL. HDLs are by far the smallest of the lipoproteins and are important for the transport of cholesterol to the liver from the periphery.

A high concentration of cholesterol (normal range 3.6–6.7mmol/l) in the plasma, in the form of lipoproteins, has been recognised as a risk factor for the development of atherosclerosis and coronary artery disease. The lipoprotein which is particularly associated with atherosclerosis is the LDL, the mechanisms being as follows. The endothelial cells that line the blood vessels normally possess LDL receptors which are involved in the clearance of the LDL from the bloodstream. If, however, the endothelial cell becomes activated, for example by injury, these receptors are destroyed and the LDL is

A high concentration of cholesterol in the plasma, in the form of lipoproteins, has been recognised as a risk factor for the development of atherosclerosis and coronary artery disease

■ *Box 5.4* Common lipid lowering drugs

Class	Agent	Proprietary name
Fibrates	Bezafibrate	Bezalip®
	Ciprofibrate	Modalim®
	Clofibrate	Atromid-S®
	Fenofibrate	Lipantil®
	Gemfibrozil	Lopid®
Statins	Atorvastatin	Lipitor®
	Cerivastatin	Lipobay®
	Fluvastatin	Lescol®
	Pravastatin	Lipostat®
	Simvastatin	Zocor®

then taken up by macrophages which migrate subendothelially to produce fatty deposits. In response to the fatty deposits there is an inflammatory response and a proliferation of smooth muscle and connective tissue cells, which form a layer over the lipid deposits. It is this cellular and protein layer that acts as a focus for the development of the thrombosis characteristic of coronary artery disease.

Drugs that decrease plasma LDL have been shown to prevent or slow the development of the atheromatous plaques which precipitate ischaemic heart disease and, in some cases, to reverse the process of atheroma development. These drugs are used in individuals who are at risk of coronary heart disease due to the presence of other risk factors, but they are normally only used in combination with other measures, such as the cessation of smoking and adherence to a strict diet. The lipid-lowering drugs can be divided into the HMG-CoA reductase inhibitors, the anion-exchange resins, the fibrates, nicotinic acid and fish oils.

5.4.2.1 HMG-CoA reductase inhibitors

The rate-limiting step in the synthesis of cholesterol depends on the conversion of 3-hydroxy-3-methoxyglutaryl-coenzyme A (HMG-CoA) to mevalonic acid by the enzyme HMG-CoA reductase. Members of a class of drugs called the statins (Box 5.4) have been shown to be selective inhibitors of this enzyme, resulting in a decreased hepatic synthesis of cholesterol. Corollaries of this effect are an increase in the synthesis of LDL receptors, increased clearance of LDL and a decrease in plasma cholesterol concentrations. In clinical use these drugs have been shown to be effective in reducing the incidence of ischaemic heart disease and myocardial infarction.

5.4.2.2 Anion-exchange resins

These agents, for example cholestyramine (colestyramine; Questran®) and colestipol (Colestiol®), are taken orally but they are not absorbed and they remain in the gut where they combine with bile salts to prevent their reabsorption. As absorption of bile salts is a major source of cholesterol, these drugs cause a reduction in plasma LDL, which in turn causes an increase in the number of LDL receptors. Clinical studies have shown that the drugs are effective in reducing the incidence of coronary heart disease but they do have associated adverse effects, such as causing gastrointestinal disturbances and reducing the absorption of fat-soluble vitamins.

5.4.2.3 The fibrates

The fibrates (Box 5.4) stimulate the actions of lipoprotein lipase and therefore accelerate the breakdown of chylomicons and VLDL; there is also a minor effect on LDL. In clinical trials these agents have been shown to reduce the incidence of coronary heart disease, but their tendency to cause adverse effects such as muscle toxicity (rhabdomyolysis) and gallstones has limited their use.

5.4.2.4 Nicotinic acid

Nicotinic acid is a vitamin which, like the related acipimox (Olbetam®), inhibits production of triglycerides and VLDL by the liver; there are also slight effects on LDL. These drugs do lower plasma cholesterol with continued use, and have been shown to reduce mortality, but their use is associated with a range of adverse effects associated with vasodilatation, for example flushing and palpitations, and with gastrointestinal disturbances.

5.4.2.5 Fish oils

It has been suggested that diets rich in fish oils decrease the incidence of heart disease, although this association is unproven. Ingestion of fish oils reduces plasma triglyceride concentrations, but increases plasma cholesterol, which would be unlikely to be beneficial in the prevention of heart disease; however, because the fish oils contain unsaturated fatty acids which can enter the synthetic pathway for prostaglandins (Chapter 9), there may be beneficial effects on platelet aggregation and the inflammatory process.

Ingestion of fish oils reduces plasma triglyceride concentrations, but increases plasma cholesterol

■ SUMMARY

- There are several disorders of the blood that can be prevented or treated by drug therapy, the first being the anaemias, in which erythrocytes lose the ability to transport oxygen. Anaemias can be caused either by a deficiency of iron, which can be treated by iron supplementation, or a deficiency of vitamin B_{12} or folic acid. The latter megaloblastic anaemias can be treated by injection of the missing nutrient. Disorders of white blood cell formation may be amenable to treatment with colony-stimulating factors.

- Disorders of haemostasis may be manifested as haemophilia, which can be treated by administration of the appropriate clotting factor, or as inappropriate blood clotting – thrombosis. Thrombotic disorders can be prevented by use of drugs to prevent platelet activation or drugs that interfere with the normal blood clotting cascade, for example warfarin or heparin. Survival of thrombotic events may be increased by prompt use of fibrinolytic agents such as streptokinase.

- The composition of the plasma component of the blood may be controlled using diuretic drugs. These act on the kidney to influence the reabsorption of ions such as sodium, potassium and chloride, and in doing so influence the urine volume and plasma volume. There are several sites within the kidney tubule at which these agents act, for example the Na^+, K^+, Cl^- transporter of the loop of Henle and the aldosterone receptor of the distal tubule. Diuretic drugs are used to reduce oedema and to reduce blood pressure in hypertension.

- The final components of the blood that may be manipulated pharmacologically are the lipoproteins. Lipids are transported within the blood as lipid particles within a protein shell, these may be large (chylomicrons) or very small (high-density lipoproteins). There is evidence that the incidence of coronary heart disease is related to blood concentrations of low-density lipoproteins (LDL) and in patients with other risk factors it has been shown that the incidence of coronary heart disease can be reduced by reduction of LDL. The mechanisms by which drugs may reduce LDL–cholesterol concentrations include inhibition of the enzyme HMG-CoA reductase, prevention of reabsorption of bile salts and stimulation of lipoprotein lipase.

■ REVISION QUESTIONS

For each question select the most appropriate answer. Correct answers are presented in Appendix 1.

1. Daily, low-dose aspirin therapy is used in prevention of platelet aggregation because:
   (a) more frequent use of low-dose aspirin causes severe adverse effects;
   (b) the irreversible effect of the aspirin lasts for the lifetime of the platelet;
   (c) aspirin has a very long plasma half-life;
   (d) frequent use causes increased activity of cyclo-oxygenase;
   (e) the effects of thromboxane A_2 last for the lifetime of the platelet.

2. Warfarin prevents coagulation by:
   (a) chelating calcium ions;
   (b) inhibiting the actions of factors IX, X, XI and XII;
   (c) stimulating plasminogen;
   (d) preventing the synthesis of factors II, VII, IX and X;
   (e) stimulating fibrinogen.

3. Heparin prevents coagulation by:
   (a) chelating calcium ions;
   (b) inhibiting the actions of factors IX, X, XI and XII;
   (c) stimulating plasminogen;
   (d) preventing the synthesis of factors II, VII, IX and X;
   (e) stimulating fibrinogen.

4. Fibrinolytic drugs are used to:
   (a) prevent clot breakdown in the treatment of menorrhagia;
   (b) prevent blood coagulation during surgery;
   (c) prevent coronary thrombosis;
   (d) remove the blood clot following coronary thrombosis;
   (e) remove the blood clot following surgery.

5. Thiazide diuretics act by:
   (a) preventing sodium reabsorption in the glomerulus;
   (b) preventing sodium reabsorption in the proximal convoluted tubule;
   (c) preventing sodium reabsorption in the loop of Henle;
   (d) preventing sodium reabsorption in the distal convoluted tubule;
   (e) preventing sodium reabsorption in the collecting duct.

6. The 'statin' lipid-lowering drugs act by:
   (a) preventing absorption of dietary fats;
   (b) preventing absorption of bile salts;
   (c) preventing synthesis of cholesterol;
   (d) stimulating cholesterol metabolism;
   (e) stimulating cholesterol excretion.

■ SELECTED READING

Galbraith, A., Bullock, S., Manias, E., Hunt, B. and Richards, A. (1999) Anticoagulant, thrombolytic and antiplatelet drugs. In Galbraith, A., Bullock, S., Manias, E., Hunt, B. and Richards, A. *Fundamentals of Pharmacology*, (Harlow: Addison Wesley Longman), 399–412.

Galbraith, A., Bullock, S., Manias, E., Hunt, B. and Richards, A. (1999) Diuretics and other renal drugs. In Galbraith, A., Bullock, S., Manias, E., Hunt, B. and Richards, A. *Fundamentals of Pharmacology*, (Harlow: Addison Wesley Longman), 413–420.

Martini, F.H. (1998) Blood. In Martini, F.H. *Fundamentals of Anatomy and Physiology* (Fourth edition), (New Jersey: Prentice Hall), 641–671.

Martini, F.H. (1998) Fluid, electrolyte, acid–base balance. In Martini, F.H. *Fundamentals of Anatomy and Physiology* (Fourth edition), (New Jersey: Prentice Hall), 1006–1036.

McDonald, R.H. (1998) Lipid-lowering drugs and atherosclerosis. In Brody, T.M., Larner, J. and Minneman, K.P. (eds) *Human Pharmacology: Molecular to Clinical* (Third edition), (St. Louis: Mosby), 279–296.

Rang, H.P., Dale, M.M. and Ritter, J.M. (1999) Atherosclerosis and lipoprotein metabolism. In Rang, H.P., Dale, M.M. and Ritter, J.M. *Pharmacology* (Fourth edition), (Edinburgh: Churchill Livingstone), 301–309.

Rang, H.P., Dale, M.M. and Ritter, J.M. (1999) Haemostasis and thrombosis. In Rang, H.P., Dale, M.M. and Ritter, J.M. *Pharmacology* (Fourth edition), (Edinburgh: Churchill Livingstone), 310–327.

Rang, H.P., Dale, M.M. and Ritter, J.M. (1999) The haemopoietic system. In Rang, H.P., Dale, M.M. and Ritter, J.M. *Pharmacology* (Fourth edition), (Edinburgh: Churchill Livingstone), 328–337.

THE TREATMENT OF RESPIRATORY DISORDERS

■ 6.1 INTRODUCTION

Ten per cent of all prescription drugs are for the treatment of disorders of the respiratory system

Diseases of the respiratory system are some of the most common, and most trouble-some, yet it is surprising that there is only a very small number of drugs which are used to treat these conditions. Despite the small number of drugs used, however, 10% of all prescription drugs are for the treatment of disorders of the respiratory system.

Probably the most common respiratory conditions requiring drug therapy are upper respiratory tract infections: coughs, colds, bronchitis, etc. Supermarket shelves are laden with remedies for these conditions, but very few of them have any effect on the course of the disease, although some may relieve some of the symptoms. The common cold is caused by at least 40 different types of virus, and as yet there are no therapeutic agents which are able to combat these viruses. This fact underlies the view that colds should not be treated with antibiotic agents because they are ineffective, this being said, however, antibiotics are sometimes administered to prevent conditions such as bronchitis which may arise as a result of a secondary bacterial infection in an individual compromised by a viral infection.

This chapter will cover drugs used to relieve the symptoms of infections (e.g. coughs), and the drugs used to treat non-infective respiratory disorders, it will not discuss the mechanisms of action nor the choice of antibiotics.

■ 6.2 THE PHYSIOLOGICAL CONTROL OF RESPIRATION

The term respiration is used to describe both the exchange of gases that occurs within the lung and the exchange and utilisation of gases at the cellular level. This chapter will only consider the effects of drugs on the processes responsible for gaseous exchange within the lung: breathing.

Normal respiration is an unconscious sequence of events but it can be controlled at will

Normal respiration is an unconscious sequence of events with rhythmic inspira-tions and expirations, but unlike autonomic functions such as gastric motility and blood pressure, respiration rate can be controlled at will. It is therefore possible to hold one's breath temporarily or to over-ventilate deliberately. Respiration is normally controlled by the inspiratory centre and the expiratory centre of the medulla; it is assumed that the inspiratory centre predominates. These centres receive input from a variety of sources, such as other brain areas, but also from chemosensors both in the brain and in the periphery. The most important factor in driving respiration is blood concentration of carbon dioxide. An increase in blood carbon dioxide is detected by chemosensors in the medulla and also in the carotid bodies and aorta, with the result that respiration rate is increased. The opposite effect occurs if blood carbon dioxide concentrations decrease, to the extent that active over-breathing may result in a temporary cessation of breathing: apnoea.

Blood pH is also monitored at the carotid bodies and aortic arch. Any decrease in blood pH results in an increase in respiration rate. In most cases the decrease in pH is a consequence of increase carbon dioxide concentrations, but other factors that decrease blood pH, for example aspirin overdose, also increase the rate of respiration.

Blood oxygen concentrations have little influence on respiration rate. Provided that the blood oxygen concentration is above a certain limit, it is the carbon dioxide concentrations that drive respiration rate. Only at exceptionally low concentrations of oxygen is there an increase in respiration rate. The decreased oxygen is detected by chemosensors in the aorta and carotid bodies, which results in stimulation of the inspiratory centre, this is seen as an emergency secondary back-up system.

In addition to these mechanisms of control for the respiratory system there are also other processes associated with the autonomic nervous system. As described in Chapter 2, the autonomic nervous system is responsible for involuntary features such as heart rate and gut motility. The lung receives input from the parasympathetic nervous system, which utilizes acetylcholine as its transmitter, but does not have direct sympathetic innervation. The lungs do, however, possess adrenoceptors and can therefore respond to circulating adrenaline. The effect of the autonomic nervous system on the respiratory system is only really important at times of 'abnormality'. An example of such an 'abnormality' would be stress, when the increased sympathetic activity results in dilation of the bronchioles and therefore increased gaseous exchange.

The effect of the autonomic nervous system on the respiratory system is only really important at times of 'abnormality' such as stress

The lungs also have mechanisms to deal with such 'abnormal' events as the inhalation of noxious substances. Noxious substances such as tobacco smoke and allergens cause bronchoconstriction via the release of agents such as acetylcholine, histamine from mast cells, leukotrienes and prostaglandins. All of these mediators induce bronchoconstriction and therefore limit the amount of the noxious substance inhaled and thus the extent of the damage caused.

■ 6.2.1 DISORDERS OF THE RESPIRATORY SYSTEM

Disorders of the respiratory system may be either chronic or acute or reoccurring and they may be due to restriction or obstruction of inspiration or to a disorder of expiration. Emphysema is a condition in which the walls of the alveoli become compromised, this causes several adjacent alveoli to fuse. The compromised alveolar walls also lose elasticity: the total picture is therefore one of accumulation of static air within large air spaces with poor vascularisation. The result is poor gaseous exchange; the patients report difficulty with breathing out and hypoxia may develop. Related disorders are those lung diseases induced by asbestos or coal dust. In these conditions the tissues become damaged and are replaced with scar tissue. Scar tissue is neither elastic, nor does it permit easy gaseous exchange, the patient therefore reports difficulty breathing (inspiration) and a greatly decreased tolerance to activity.

Chronic obstructive pulmonary disease (COPD) describes a progressive, irreversible condition characterised by airway obstruction. In some cases the obstruction is due to bronchoconstriction, often induced by inhalation of noxious chemicals, or is due to hypersecretion of bronchial secretions such as mucus. In both cases there is long-term irreversible tissue damage.

Chronic obstructive pulmonary disease (COPD) is a progressive, irreversible condition, the most common cause of which is smoking

Asthma is a chronic condition in which there are periods of reversible airway obstruction. Typically the sufferer has intermittent attacks of breathlessness (dyspnoea) and coughing, which are triggered by stimuli not normally considered to be noxious. Common examples of such stimuli are allergens such as grass pollens, cold air and irritant fumes. Up to 10% of the population suffers from asthma, although there are wide variations across different countries. Some authorities suggest that an increase in the prevalence and severity of asthma accompanies industrialisation and an increase in pollution, whereas others believe that other factors are more important: New Zealand, for example, is relatively under-industrialized but has a high incidence of asthma. Some people certainly have a genetic predisposition to asthma, indicating a predisposition to bronchoconstriction in response to certain stimuli, but it should also be noted that the reports of increased prevalence of asthma in developed countries may reflect increased awareness and likelihood of diagnosis.

Most 'asthmatic attacks' are characterised by two phases: the first phase is the transient bronchoconstriction which occurs following exposure of the hypersensitive individual to the trigger. This first phase is short lived. The second phase onsets about 4 hours after the initial exposure, is more profound than the initial phase and may last for several hours. Nearly all forms of asthma exhibit the two phases, but they may be closely sequential so that there is no apparent, early, improvement of the symptoms; there may also be multiple insults so that there is a chain of initial and secondary phases. The first phase of the asthmatic attack is probably due to the short-lived bronchospasm induced by released histamine, leukotrienes and prostaglandins. The late phase is a slowly developing inflammatory response. Even if the symptoms of the first phase are masked, for example by use of bronchodilators (Section 6.3.4), the second phase of the condition ensues, resulting in a slow accumulation of the deleterious effects of the inflammation.

In most cases, asthma is not life-threatening, and if correctly controlled, has limited effects on quality of life. It must be remembered, however, that severe asthma attacks (status asthmaticus) may take several days to reverse and can prove fatal.

Approximately 10% of the population suffers from asthma

In most cases asthma is not life-threatening but severe asthma attacks can prove fatal

■ 6.3 DRUGS AFFECTING THE RESPIRATORY SYSTEM
6.3.1 RESPIRATORY STIMULANTS

Some conditions such as brain damage, drug overdose and profound anaesthesia may cause acute respiratory failure. In most cases the condition results in death, but in some cases administration of a respiratory stimulant may be of use. The only currently available respiratory stimulant is doxapram, although nikethamide has been used previously. The mechanism of action of these drugs is unknown, but they may act on the chemosensors of the carotid body and aorta to stimulate breathing. These drugs also act as central nervous stimulants and therefore have a tendency to induce convulsions, which may make the patient's predicament worse.

■ 6.3.2 RESPIRATORY DEPRESSANTS

As stated in Chapter 3, many centrally acting depressants have the effect of depressing respiration. The most notable of these are the opioids, such as heroin and morphine, where respiratory depression is the primary cause of death following overdose. In such cases there are no physical obstructions to breathing, but because of the CNS depression there is no respiratory drive: the individual does not feel the need to breathe.

There is only one therapeutic indication for respiratory depression: cough suppression. Cough is an involuntary response to the presence of foreign matter in the trachea or bronchi. Coughing is brought about by contraction of the expiratory muscle while the

■ *Box 6.1* The constituents of some common cough remedies

Classification	Active ingredient	Proprietary name
Cough suppressant	Codeine	Galcodine®
	Pholcodine	Galenphol®
Expectorant	Ammonium chloride	Benylin Chesty Cough®
	Guaiphenesin	Venos for Dry Coughs®
	(guaifenesin)	Robitussin Chesty Cough®
Demulcent	Glycerol	Nirolex Dry Cough Linctus®
	Honey	Vicks Vaposyrup for
		Tickly Coughs®

glottis and epiglottis are closed. Sudden relaxation of the glottis and epiglottis allow the escape of pressurised gas, taking with it the foreign body. Like breathing, cough is an automatic response, but it can be consciously suppressed and there can be voluntary coughs. Cough is believed to be mediated by a group of cells in the medulla called the cough centre, these cells are probably related, in some way, to the respiratory centres.

In the same way that opioids can inhibit respiration, they also suppress the cough reflex. This removes the symptom of the cough, but does not address the underlying disease, for example infection or carcinoma. The most commonly used opioid cough suppressants are codeine and dextromethorphan (Box 6.1).

In the same way that opioids can inhibit respiration, they also suppress the cough reflex

Other than the opioid cough suppressants, few, if any, of the other cough medications have clinically proven efficacy. Expectorant cough medications contain irritants such as amonium chloride or ipecacuanha, the rationale behind these remedies is that they promote bronchial secretions, increase the volume of the bronchial fluids and therefore facilitate expectoration. The demulcent cough medications which contain syrup and glycerol are given to lubricate the throat and therefore soothe a dry cough.

■ 6.3.3 SURFACTANTS

Normally if two tissues come into contact with each other, they adhere together. It would be rational, therefore, to expect the small chambers of the lung, alveoli, to collapse at the end of expiration, and for the two surfaces to adhere. Under normal circumstances this does not occur; first, because the lung does not empty completely, there is a residual volume of about 1 litre out of a total lung volume of about 6 litres, and, secondly because of the presence of lung surfactant. Lung surfactant is normally produced by the cells of the alveoli and acts to prevent alveolar adhesions. In the fetus, however, there is no need for lung surfactant prior to birth because oxygen and nutrients are obtained via the placenta. Production of lung surfactant does not begin until about the last week of pregnancy (week 40), in time for the normal transition to obtaining the oxygen via the lungs. In the premature neonate this absence of surfactant may give rise to respiratory difficulty: infant respiratory distress syndrome. One practice used to overcome this deficiency is to provide the baby with pressurised gas containing a high oxygen concentration. The high pressure acts to open the alveoli while the raised oxygen supports respiration. A new development is the production of synthetic lung surfactants such as beractant (Survanta®) and colfosceril palmitate (Exosurf Neonatal®), which are administered via an endotrachial tube. These new treatments have been shown to be highly effective in the relief of infant respiratory distress syndrome in premature neonates.

Adult respiratory distress syndrome occurs when the secretion of surfactant is compromised or the surfactant is removed. Any form of alveolar oedema may induce respiratory distress syndrome. Conditions that may induce it include inhalation of fluids such as water or inhalation of noxious fumes. In some cases these patients may be treated by administration of the synthetic surfactants.

■ 6.3.4 BRONCHODILATORS

The first-line treatment of asthma is usually the use of bronchodilators. These drugs physiologically antagonise the bronchoconstriction of the early phase of the asthma, and may act for a sufficient duration to relieve the second phase. The benefit of these agents is that they bring immediate relief of the breathlessness; they do not, however, prevent the inflammatory stage and any possible consequential long-term tissue damage. It is generally believed that infrequent asthma attacks can be treated with bronchodilators, but that additional forms of treatment should be used if the attacks become more regular, see Section 6.3.5.

Chronic obstructive airways disease (COPD) may also respond to bronchodilators. As stated in Section 6.2.1, COPD is said to be an irreversible condition, but there must be a reversible component as use of bronchodilators has been shown to provide some symptomatic relief.

Bronchodilators can be divided into three classes: β-adrenoceptor agonists, muscarinic receptor antagonists and xanthines.

6.3.4.1 β-Adrenoceptor agonists

As described in Chapter 2 the bronchioles possess β-adrenoceptors that are qualitatively different from those found on the heart. Cardiac β-adrenoceptors are designated β_1, and those on the bronchioles are β_2. It has been known for many years that administration of catecholamines such as adrenaline and noradrenaline induce bronchodilation and an increase in the rate and force of contraction of the heart, but it was only with the development of the selective β_2-adrenoceptor antagonists that bronchodilation could be achieved without the cardiac effects. The most commonly used β_2-adrenoceptor agonist is salbutamol, usually administered in the form of an inhaler, although it can be administered in tablet form, as a syrup or via several other methods to effect delivery directly to the bronchioles. It is generally assumed that the local, targetted delivery of the drug to the lung results in fewer systemic side-effects, but there are sometimes difficulties in administering inhalation therapies during an acute episode of asthma.

> β-Adrenoceptor agonists such as salbutamol are the most commonly used bronchodilating agents in the treatment of asthma

The adverse effects of the β_2-adrenoceptor agonists all relate to effects on receptors other than those in the lungs, thus there may be peripheral vasodilation, headache and tremor. Non-selective effects on β_1-adrenoceptors may result in tachycardia, but this is rare when the drug is given by inhalation.

Salmeterol is a long-acting β_2-adrenoceptor agonist which may be used by inhalation on a once daily basis, but such medication is often considered to be inappropriate in the treatment of asthma (Section 6.3.5). Salmeterol does have a place, however, in the treatment of COPD, and for the relief of nocturnal asthma, where the patient may take the drug before retiring in order to prevent asthma that may occur in the early hours of the morning. A list of commonly used β_2-adrenoceptor agonists is presented in Box 6.2.

6.3.4.2 Muscarinic receptor antagonists

The β_2-adrenoceptor agonists produce bronchodilation by mimicking the effect of sympathetic stimulation on the bronchioles. The converse is to inhibit the bronchoconstrictory

■ *Box 6.2* Selective β_2-adrenoceptor agonists used for the relief of asthma and chronic obstructive airways disease

Active ingredient	Proprietary name	Properties
Salbutamol	Ventolin®	Injection, tablets, syrup or inhaler; short acting
Terbutaline	Bricanyl®	Tablets, syrup or inhaler; short acting
Fenoterol	Berotec®	Inhaler; short acting
Salmeterol	Serevent®	Inhaler; slow onset, long duration of action
Eformoterol	Foradil®	Inhaler; slow onset, long duration of action
	Oxis®	Inhaler; slow onset, long duration of action

■ *Box 6.3* Xanthines used in the relief of asthma

Xanthine	Proprietary name
Theophylline	Nuelin®
	Lasma®
	Slo-Phyllin®
	Theo-Dur®
	Uniphyllin Continus®
Aminophylline	Phyllocontin Continus®

effects of the parasympathetic nervous system, thereby inducing bronchodilation. The antimuscarinic agents of choice are ipratropium (Atrovent®) and oxitropium (Oxivent®) as these agents do not cross the blood–brain barrier and are poorly absorbed. These agents are used in the form of an inhaler to induce bronchodilation but have less likelihood of inducing the side-effects typical of other anticholinergic agents.

Ipratropium and oxitropium may be used to treat asthma, but they are often seen as being the bronchodilators of choice for the treatment of COPD because of their inhibitory effects on the secretion of bronchial fluids.

6.3.4.3 Xanthines

Xanthines such as caffeine, theophylline and theobromine are present in tea, coffee and cocoa. These and related agents (Box 6.3) are, however, all of use in the relief of asthma, although they are less effective than the β_2-adrenoceptor agonists. The mechanism of action remains unclear, but several effects are well documented; the best-known action being inhibition of phosphodiesterase. Phosphodiesterase is the enzyme responsible for the breakdown of cyclic adenosine monophosphate (cAMP), thus inhibition of its actions prolongs the effects of cAMP. As described in Chapter 1, cAMP is a second messenger for several G-protein coupled receptors, the effects of the xanthines therefore are to enhance or mimic the effects of the natural agonists on these receptors. The natural second messenger for β_2-adrenoceptors is cAMP, thus in the case of asthma, the xanthines may be acting by potentiating or mimicking the effects of β_2-adrenoceptor agonists. Potentiation of cAMP may also reduce the severity of the inflammatory events that occur during the later phase of an asthmatic attack.

Many xanthines also antagonise receptors for adenosine, but it is unlikely that this is the mechanism by which they are able to relieve asthma.

When used therapeutically, xanthines are given in either liquid or tablet form, often as a sustained release formulation which allows a twice daily dosing schedule. The adverse effects of the xanthines are related to their non-selective mechanism of action, thus there is central nervous system stimulation, which may result in insomnia and even convulsions; there are inotropic and chronotropic effects on the heart, resulting in palpitations and tachycardia, and there are mild diuretic effects on the kidney. The most frequently reported adverse effects are the feelings of nausea and gastrointestinal disturbance. It should also be noted that the therapeutic margin for theophylline is very small, thus a small overdose may result in toxicity, it is because of this that plasma concentrations of theophylline are frequently monitored.

■ 6.3.5 OTHER ANTI-ASTHMATICS

Steroid inhalers do not relieve asthma but they prevent both the initial and the later phase

Bronchodilating agents are effective in the relief of the initial phase of asthma but they offer no protection against the damage induced by the later inflammatory phase. It is because of this that clinicians now realise that anti-inflammatory agents are the correct form of treatment for asthma that requires regular (daily) treatment with bronchodilating agents. The mechanisms of action of the anti-inflammatory agents are presented in Chapter 9. These agents do not relieve an ongoing asthma attack, but they are effective in its prevention, thus they prevent the initial response that leads to the bronchoconstriction and they prevent the later inflammatory events. The most commonly used anti-inflammatory agents in the treatment of asthma are the steroids (Chapter 9 and Box 6.4), which are usually administered in the form of an inhaler in order to reduce the risks of systemic side-effects (Chapters 8 and 9). Chronic obstructive airways disease does not respond to steroid therapy.

A newer form of treatment involves the inhibitors of the cysteinyl leukotrienes, inflammatory mediators which act on the leukotriene C_4 receptor (Chapter 9). These agents, montelukast (Singulair®) and zafirlukast (Accolate®), are administered orally either once or twice daily and have been shown to be effective in the prevention of both phases of asthma, including exercise-induced asthma.

■ *Box 6.4* Inhaled corticosteroids for the treatment of asthma

Corticosteroid	Proprietary name
Beclomethasone	AeroBec®
(beclometasone)	Asmabec®
	Becotide®
	Becloforte®
	Qvar®
Budesonide	Pulmicort®
Fluticasone	Flixotide®

■ SUMMARY

- Diseases of the respiratory system are some of the most common and most troublesome, with 10% of all prescription drugs being used to treat respiratory disorders, but there are only a few important classes of pharmacological agents which are used for their effects on the lungs.

- Respiratory stimulants and respiratory depressants act on the central nervous system to enhance or suppress respiration, respectively. The respiratory stimulants are used only in cases such as drug overdose or brain damage, and because of their stimulant effects on the brain there is an accompanying risk of inducing convulsions. The only respiratory suppressants used therapeutically are the opioid agonists, which are used as cough suppressants. An overdose of an opioid agonist may result in fatal respiratory suppression.

- Asthma and chronic obstructive pulmonary disease (COPD) are two common conditions characterised by difficulty with breathing. In many cases the symptoms may be relieved by use of bronchodilating agents such as β_2-adrenoceptor agonists, muscarinic antagonists or xanthines. These agents are effective in reversing the initial bronchoconstriction phase of asthma and the reversible element of COPD, but they do not prevent the long-term damage induced by the later inflammatory phase of asthma. The mechanism of action of the xanthines is unclear, but they may act by enhancing the effects of cAMP and therefore mimicking the effects of β_2-adrenoceptor agonists. The adverse effects of β_2-adrenoceptor agonists and muscarinic antagonists are reduced by targetted delivery to the lungs by aerosol inhalers; xanthines are administered orally and their use is accompanied by the risk of toxicity.

- The most appropriate therapy for severe asthma is prophylactic steroid therapy, again usually by inhaler. This form of therapy prevents the initial bronchoconstrictory phase as well as inhibiting the later inflammatory phase and the associated risk of long-term damage.

- A newer form of treatment involves inhibitors of the cysteinyl leukotrienes which have been shown to be effective in the prevention of both phases of asthma, including exercise-induced asthma.

■ REVISION QUESTIONS

For each question select the most appropriate answer. Correct answers are presented in Appendix 1.

1. Salbutamol relieves the symptoms of asthma by:
   - (a) stimulation of muscarinic receptors;
   - (b) antagonism of muscarinic receptors;
   - (c) stimulation of β_2-adrenoceptors;
   - (d) antagonism of β_2-adrenoceptors;
   - (e) stimulation of β_1-adrenoceptors.

2. Atrovent® relieves the symptoms of chronic obstructive pulmonary disease by:
   - (a) stimulation of muscarinic receptors;
   - (b) antagonism of muscarinic receptors;
   - (c) stimulation of β_2-adrenoceptors;
   - (d) antagonism of β_2-adrenoceptors;
   - (e) stimulation of β_1-adrenoceptors.

3. Codeine relieves cough by:
   (a) promoting bronchial secretions, therefore facilitating expectoration;
   (b) lubricating the throat;
   (c) relaxing the smooth muscles of the bronchi;
   (d) suppressing the cough centre;
   (e) suppressing the respiratory centre.

4. Ipratropium and oxitropium are used as bronchodilators in preference to other agents that act on the same receptors because:
   (a) they are rapidly excreted by the kidney, unchanged;
   (b) they produce a long-lasting effect;
   (c) they are poorly absorbed and do not cross the blood–brain barrier;
   (d) they are selective for the receptors concerned;
   (e) they are non-competitive antagonists.

5. The most appropriate treatment for frequent sufferers of asthma is:
   (a) inhaled β-adrenoceptor agonists;
   (b) inhaled β-adrenoceptor antagonists;
   (c) inhaled muscarinic agonists;
   (d) inhaled xanthines;
   (e) inhaled corticosteroids.

6. Salbutamol is commonly used for the relief of acute asthma because:
   (a) it prevents the long-term deleterious effects of asthma;
   (b) it is free from adverse effects;
   (c) it provides rapid relief;
   (d) it prevents the development of asthma;
   (e) it is the cheapest form of therapy.

■ SELECTED READING

Galbraith, A., Bullock, S., Manias, E., Hunt, B. and Richards, A. (1999) Bronchodilators, inhaled corticosteroids, respiratory stimulants, oxygen therapy, asthma prophylactics and surfactants. In Galbraith, A., Bullock, S., Manias, E., Hunt, B. and Richards, A. *Fundamentals of Pharmacology*, (Harlow: Addison Wesley Longman), 456–467.

Martini, F.H. (1998) The respiratory system. In Martini, F.H. *Fundamentals of anatomy and physiology*, (Fourth edition), (New Jersey: Prentice Hall), 814–860.

Murphey, A.W. and Platts-Mills T.A.E. (1998) Drugs used in asthma and obstructive lung disease. In Brody, T.M., Larner, J. and Minneman, K.P. (eds) *Human Pharmacology: Molecular to Clinical* (Third edition), (St. Louis: Mosby), 797–810.

Rang, H.P., Dale, M.M. and Ritter, J.M. (1999) The respiratory system. In Rang, H.P., Dale, M.M. and Ritter, J.M. *Pharmacology* (Fourth edition), (Edinburgh: Churchill Livingstone), 338–350.

■ COMPUTER-AIDED LEARNING PACKAGE

Further details of these learning packages can be found at
http://cbl.leeds.ac.uk/raven/pha/phCAL.html

The Pharmacology of Asthma (version 1.96), Pharma-CAL-ogy, British Pharmacological Society, University of Leeds.

DRUGS ACTING ON THE GASTROINTESTINAL TRACT, BLADDER AND UTERUS

■ 7.1 INTRODUCTION

The gastrointestinal tract, bladder and uterus are considered together in a single chapter primarily because they are all smooth-muscle organs. The function of the gastrointestinal tract is to process foodstuffs such that they are broken down to their component parts, for example amino acids, carbohydrates and lipids, and to enable absorption of the component parts. It is also important in the excretion of non-water-soluble products of metabolism, for example bile salts. These functions are achieved by the regular, ordered movement of the foodstuffs through different areas of the gut, each area being responsible for a different aspect of digestion. The gastric acid and pepsins of the stomach, for example, are responsible for the digestion of proteins, whereas the enzymes and bile salts within the duodenum digest both carbohydrates and polysaccharides and facilitate emulsification of fats. Effective digestion, absorption and excretion requires regulation of the rate of transit of the gut contents such that the appropriate enzymes are secreted only when foodstuffs are present, the enzymes are allowed sufficient time to act before the contents are moved on to the next area of the gut and there is sufficient time for absorption to occur. Any dysfunction of gut motility, such as diarrhoea or constipation, disrupts digestion, absorption and excretion, which, in turn, may have more widespread effects on the health and well-being of the individual. It is because of these fears, and because of the discomfort and inconvenience of even minor disorders of the gastrointestinal tract, that drugs which act on the gastrointestinal tract are amongst the most frequently used forms of medicine, particularly amongst those who self-medicate.

The discomfort and inconvenience of even minor disorders of the gastrointestinal tract means that laxatives and antidiarrhoeals are some of the most commonly used medications

The bladder, like the gut, is comprised of smooth muscle and is therefore not under voluntary control. It is therefore necessary sometimes to use drugs to either induce or inhibit bladder contractions.

The third smooth muscle organ to be considered in this chapter is the uterus. In terms of therapeutics, the most important aspect of the uterus is its role in pregnancy. Uterine contractions are influenced by a large number of factors, for example female reproductive hormones, locally produced prostaglandins and the sympathetic nervous system. All of these factors must interact to ensure that uterine contractions do not expel the embryo or fetus early in pregnancy, but do expel the fetus at full term. In some cases pharmacological intervention is required in order to facilitate the delivery of a healthy baby, by either inhibiting inappropriate uterine contractions or by initiating contractions.

Drugs acting on the non-pregnant uterus may be of use in the relief of period pain

Drugs acting on the non-pregnant uterus may also be of use in the relief of dysmenor-rhoea (painful menstrual periods).

■ 7.2 DRUGS ACTING ON THE GASTROINTESTINAL TRACT
7.2.1 THE PHYSIOLOGY OF THE GASTROINTESTINAL TRACT

An understanding of the physiology of the control of gastric acid secretion, enzyme secretion and gut motility has facilitated the development of drugs for the treatment of such conditions as gastric and duodenal ulceration, diarrhoea and constipation. The activity of the gastrointestinal tract is influenced by the activity of the sympathetic and parasympathetic nervous systems, although co-ordinated gut activity is achieved prim-arily by the secretion of local gastrointestinal hormones (figure 7.1). As the food enters the stomach there is secretion of gastrin, which not only initiates secretion of gastric acid but also stimulates gastric and intestinal motility and induces relaxation of the pyloric sphincter. In readiness for the passage of food into the duodenum, gastrin causes secre-tion of digestive juices from the pancreas and the contraction of the gall bladder, result-ing in the mixture of bile salts with the gut contents. Gastrin also promotes the growth of gastric and intestinal mucosa for the repair of any damage that may have occurred to these cells following exposure to gastric acid and digestive enzymes.

By the time the food enters the duodenum an alkaline environment has been achieved by the prior secretion of pancreatic juices. The passage of food into the duodenum results in the secretion of cholecystokinin and secretin, which ensure the continued secretion of bile salts and pancreatic enzymes into the gut lumen; cholecystokinin also inhibits the motility of the now-empty stomach and causes contraction of the pyloric sphincter to prevent retrograde passage of gut contents.

As the partially digested food passes out of the duodenum and into the jejunum and ileum the secretion of digestive juices by the intestinal mucosa is stimulated by gastric inhibitory peptide, which also inhibits further secretion of gastric acid. The presence within the gut of products of digestion then causes secretion of somatostatin, which inhibits release of all digestive juices. The final stage is the secretion of motilin as the duodenum empties and as the pH returns to 4.5. Motilin causes slow peristaltic contractions of the whole

• **Figure 7.1** An illustration of the role of gastrointestinal hormones in the co-ordination of gastrointestinal tract function and activity (Reproduced from Gard, P.R. (1998) *Modules in Life Science: Human Endocrinology*, London: Taylor & Francis)

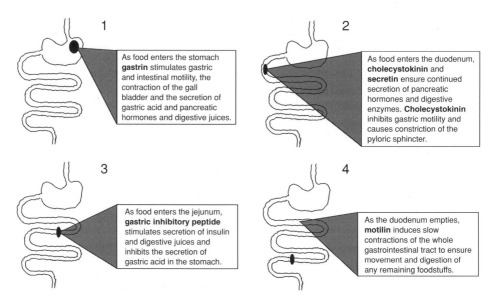

1. As food enters the stomach **gastrin** stimulates gastric and intestinal motility, the contraction of the gall bladder and the secretion of gastric acid and pancreatic hormones and digestive juices.

2. As food enters the duodenum, **cholecystokinin** and **secretin** ensure continued secretion of pancreatic hormones and digestive enzymes. **Cholecystokinin** inhibits gastric motility and causes constriction of the pyloric sphincter.

3. As food enters the jejunum, **gastric inhibitory peptide** stimulates secretion of insulin and digestive juices and inhibits the secretion of gastric acid in the stomach.

4. As the duodenum empties, **motilin** induces slow contractions of the whole gastrointestinal tract to ensure movement and digestion of any remaining foodstuffs.

gastrointestinal tract to ensure movement and digestion of any residual, undigested food-stuffs. This slow activity continues until the next arrival of food at the stomach.

■ 7.2.2 THE AETIOLOGY AND TREATMENT OF GASTRIC AND DUODENAL ULCERATION

The mucosal cells of the stomach and upper intestine are under constant attack by the digestive forces of gastric acid and pepsin. Under normal circumstances, gastric acid and pepsin are only secreted at times when there is food within the stomach, thus the digestive activity is concentrated towards the stomach contents. In addition, the gastric and duodenal mucosa have barriers which normally protect them from damage. The protective barriers are of two forms: the first is the secretion of mucus, which lies over the epithelial cells and therefore separates them from the gut contents. The second is the secretion of sodium hydrogen carbonate (sodium bicarbonate) which, because of the mucus barrier, remains trapped adjacent to the epithelial cells and therefore acts locally to neutralise the gastric acid. Any condition where there is inappropriate or excessive secretion of gastric acid, or where there is a breakdown of the protective barrier, can result in damage to the gastric or duodenal mucosa: gastric or duodenal ulcer.

Gastric acid is synthesised in the parietal cells of the stomach by the action of carbonic anhydrase, which converts hydrogen and carbon dioxide to carbonic acid; the ionisation of the carbonic acid coupled with the active transport of chloride ions results in the formation of hydrochloric acid within the stomach lumen (figure 7.2). The secretion of gastric acid is controlled by the actions of gastrin, histamine and acetylcholine. Gastrin secretion is stimulated by the presence of food in the stomach, and by acetylcholine and adrenaline. It acts on specific gastrin receptors of the parietal cells to increase the

> The stomach and upper intestine are under constant attack by the digestive forces of gastric acid and pepsin

> Inappropriate or excessive secretion of gastric acid, or a breakdown of the protective barriers, results in gastric or duodenal ulceration

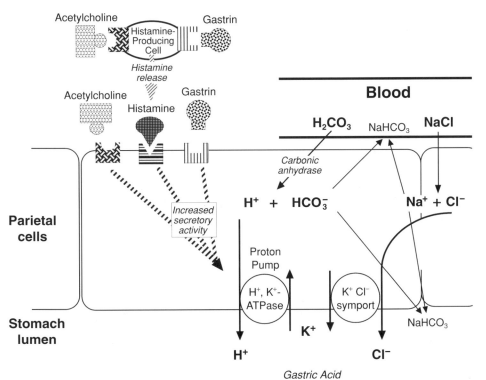

• **Figure 7.2** Factors involved in the secretion of gastric acid by the parietal cells of the stomach

mobilisation of intracellular calcium, which enhances gastric acid secretion; gastrin also acts on mast cells to enhance histamine release (see later). Acetylcholine, acting on muscarinic (M_3) receptors, which increase intracellular calcium by the opening of a ligand-gated calcium channel, also potentiates gastric acid secretion. Like gastrin, acetylcholine, acting via muscarinic (M_1) receptors, is also able to enhance histamine release.

Histamine is the most important mediator in the control of gastric acid secretion

The most important mediator in the control of gastric acid secretion is believed to be histamine. Histamine is known to act on histamine (H_2) receptors of the parietal cells and to increase gastric acid secretion via synthesis of cyclic AMP. Antagonism of the H_2 receptors decreases the acid secretion stimulated by histamine, but also decreases acid secretion stimulated by gastrin. It is now believed that the release of histamine is the most important feature of the effects of both gastrin and acetylcholine on gastric acid secretion; thus histamine is acting as an intermediary. It is clear, however, that both acetylcholine and gastrin, acting via an increase in intracellular calcium, are able to increase gastric acid secretion directly. The common end point for the actions of histamine, acetylcholine and gastrin is the stimulation of the proton pump (H^+, K^+-ATPase) of the parietal cells (figure 7.2).

Inappropriate secretion of gastric acid can occur at times of stress, presumably due to the effect of adrenaline on gastrin secretion, and in Zollinger–Ellison syndrome, which is a condition where there is a gastrin-secreting tumour. Both conditions may result in gastric or duodenal ulcers. Ulceration may also occur if the protective barrier becomes compromised. Prostaglandins E_2 and I_2 are both involved in the secretion of the mucus layer and the bicarbonate, thus drugs such as steroidal and non-steroidal anti-inflammatory agents (Chapter 9), which prevent prostaglandin synthesis, are associated with a break-down of the protective barrier and an increase in the incidence of gastric ulceration. Alcohol also disrupts the barrier. Another factor that can compromise the protective barrier is the bacterium *Helicobacter pylori*. This bacterium has been identified in the gastric and duodenal mucosa of many ulcer patients; eradication of the infection is associated with recovery from the ulcer, whereas deliberate infection with *Helicobacter* is associated with the development of ulceration.

Deliberate infection with *Helicobacter pylori* results in gastric ulceration

Treatments for gastric and duodenal ulcers can be aimed either at decreasing gastric acid secretion, enhancing the protective barrier or removing the causative agent (for example gastrin-secreting tumour or *Helicobacter pylori*).

7.2.2.1 Histamine (H_2) antagonists

Competitive antagonists of the histamine (H_2) receptor were introduced for the treatment of gastric and duodenal ulcers approximately 30 years ago. These drugs decrease the effects of histamine and therefore decrease baseline acid secretion as well as decreasing the effects of acetylcholine and gastrin (see above). The reduction of acid secretion removes the cause of the ulceration and therefore promotes healing of existing ulcers. These drugs are also used to prevent recurrence of ulceration. The major differences between the H_2 antagonists listed in Box 7.1 is the plasma half-life and therefore the dose frequency, although there are also some differences in the profiles of adverse effects. All H_2 antagonists have been associated with occasional reports of sedation and dizziness, and with some effects on the heart; these are probably associated with antagonism of H_2 receptors in the brain and heart, respectively. There have also been reports of gynaecomastia and impotence, more frequently, but not exclusively, associated with cimetidine; this effect is related to the antagonism of androgen receptors. Unlike the other available H_2 antagonists, cimetidine also inhibits some hepatic enzymes, which can result in clinically important interactions with some other medications if they are being taken concurrently.

■ *Box 7.1* Drugs used for the treatment of gastric and duodenal ulcers

Drug	*Proprietary name*
Histamine (H$_2$) antagonists	
Cimetidine	Dyspamet® (tablets)
	Tagamet® (tablets)
Famotidine	Pepcid® (tablets)
Nizatidine	Axid® (capsules, injection)
Ranitidine	Zantac® (tablets)
Acetylcholine (muscarinic) antagonist	
Pirenzepine	Gastrozepin® (tablets)
Proton pump inhibitors	
Omeprazole	Losec® (capsules)
Lansoprazole	Zoton® (capsules)

7.2.2.2 Muscarinic antagonists

Antagonists of the muscarinic acetylcholine receptors have a variety of effects on the gastrointestinal tract, constipation, for example, is a side-effect of many anticholinergic drugs. The only antimuscarinic agent available for treatment of gastric and duodenal ulcers is pirenzepine, which selectively inhibits the M$_1$-subtype of the receptor. Antagonism of the M$_1$ receptor results in a reduced histamine release and thus reduced histamine-induced gastric acid secretion; the anticholinergic effects, however, also give rise to side-effects, such as dry mouth and blurred vision, in a large proportion of patients.

7.2.2.3 Proton pump inhibitors

The newest form of anti-ulcer therapy is the proton pump inhibitors. These drugs, for example omeprazole, block the H$^+$,K$^+$-ATPase of the parietal cells and thus prevent the acid secretion stimulated by histamine, acetylcholine and gastrin.

7.2.2.4 Antacids

Probably the oldest form of treatment for gastric or duodenal ulcers is antacids, although these are more effective in the treatment of duodenal ulcers than gastric ulcers. The aim of antacid therapy is to reduce the corrosive action of the hydrochloric acid by simply neutralising the acidity, thus promoting the healing of, and relieving the pain of, the ulcer. The common forms of antacids are based on aluminium, magnesium and calcium salts, for example aluminium hydroxide and magnesium carbonate. Sucralfate is also a basic aluminium salt, but in this case it is a salt of sucrose octasulphate. Sucralfate has a slight effect on gastric pH, but is effective in promoting the healing of the ulcer; its predominant mechanisms of action are the formation of a protective 'coat' over the area of the ulcer, suppression of *Helicobacter* infection and some complexation of pepsin and bile salts.

A special case of ulcer-like condition is reflux oesophagitis. In this condition gastric contents pass in a retrograde direction from the stomach to the oesophagus, thus inducing irritation of the mucous membrane. Standard treatments for gastric and duodenal ulcers are also effective in reflux oesophagitis, but one specialized form of treatment is the combination of an antacid together with alginate. The presence of the alginate acts to retain the antacid within the oesophagus amd also to act as a protective 'coat' over the lesion.

The oldest form of treatment for gastric or duodenal ulcers is to use antacids

■ 7.2.3 THE TREATMENT OF VOMITING

Vomiting is an important function of the gastrointestinal tract that can occur in response to repulsive stimuli such as sights or smells, motion and certain toxins and drugs. Although superficially an action of the gut, vomiting involves the co-ordinated activity of the voluntary respiratory and abdominal muscles and the smooth muscles of the gastrointestinal tract. The activity of these muscles is co-ordinated by the vomiting centre of the brain. The activity of the vomiting centre is itself controlled by the chemosensory trigger zone (CTZ) of the brain. It is the chemosensory trigger zone which initiates vomiting in response to blood-borne toxins, repulsive stimuli and motion; local irritation of the gastrointestinal tract has a local effect. Neurotransmitters shown to be involved in the control of vomiting include acetylcholine, histamine, 5-hydroxytryptamine, dopamine and enkephalins, thus drugs for the relief and prevention of nausea and vomiting are directed at receptors for these neurotransmitters.

The chemosensory trigger zone initiates vomiting, a gastrointestinal event associated with repulsive sights, smells and tastes

7.2.3.1 Histamine and acetylcholine antagonists

Antagonists of the histamine (H_1) receptor or the muscarinic receptors are effective in the relief of nausea and vomiting induced by motion or by direct stimulation of the stomach (Box 7.2), but are ineffective against direct stimulation of the CTZ. It is generally believed that the antimuscarinic agents are more effective than the antihistamines; however, the anticholinergic actions of many antihistamines serve to enhance their activity.

7.2.3.2 Dopamine antagonists

The most important group of dopamine antagonists used therapeutically are the phenothiazines; these are used not only in the treatment of psychoses (Chapter 3), but also for the relief of nausea and vomiting. For the relief of nausea and vomiting these agents are effective against most stimuli of the CTZ, but are less effective against direct stimulation of the gut. Their mechanism of action probably relies on antagonism of the dopamine (D_2) receptor; however, most phenothiazines also have anticholinergic and antihistamine properties, which will add to their efficacy. Another dopamine antagonist,

---

■ *Box 7.2* Drugs used in the treatment of nausea and vomiting

Drug	Proprietary name
Muscarinic antagonist	
Hyoscine	Scopoderm® (skin patch)
Histamine antagonists	
Cinnarizine	Stugeron® (tablets)
Cyclizine	Valoid® (tablets)
Dimenhydrinate	Dramamine® (tablets)
Promethazine theoclate	Avomine® (tablets)
Prochlorperazine	Stemetil® (tablets)
Dopamine antagonists	
Domperidone	Motilium® (tablets)
Metoclopramide	Maxolon® (tablets)
5-HT antagonists	
Granisetron	Kytril® (tablets)
Ondansetron	Zofran® (tablets)

metoclopramide, is also used as an antiemetic although it has other effects on the gastrointestinal tract.

As described in Chapter 3, dopamine antagonists are associated with a range of adverse effects, for example those relating to increased secretion of prolactin (Chapter 8) and those related to disruption of the neuronal control of movement.

7.2.3.3 5-Hydroxytryptamine antagonists

5-Hydroxytryptamine (5-HT) is an important transmitter in the brain and the gut, thus 5-HT of both gut and brain origin have been shown to be important in vomiting. Antagonists of the 5-HT$_3$ receptor, such as ondansetron and granisetron, are effective antiemetics, and are used particularly for the relief of nausea and vomiting associated with treatment with anticancer (cytotoxic) agents.

7.2.3.4 Miscellaneous antiemetic agents

High doses of the glucocorticoids, dexamethasone and methylprednisolone, are effective antiemetic agents, although their mechanism of action is unknown. The cannabinoid derivative nabilone is also effective as an antiemetic, particularly in emesis related to cancer chemotherapy. Again, the mechanism of action is unknown although an action at opioid receptors may be involved.

■ 7.2.4 THE TREATMENT OF DIARRHOEA

Diarrhoea is the accelerated movement of content through the gastrointestinal tract, the most obvious feature of which is the reduced reabsorption of water in the colon, which results in the excretion of liquid or semi-liquid faeces. There are many causes of diarrhoea, ranging from toxins and infections to anxiety, and there are many consequences, ranging from inconvenience to death due to excessive loss of fluid and electrolytes. In healthy adults the usual form of treatment for acute diarrhoea is simple fluid replacement. This strategy is adopted on the grounds that the condition will be resolved more rapidly if the gut is allowed to expel the toxins or microorganism. Where the diarrhoea persists, and is proven to be of microbial or viral origin, the use of anti-infective agents may be instituted.

> There are many causes of diarrhoea, ranging from infections to anxiety, and there are many consequences, ranging from inconvenience to death

In many cases, however, non-treatment of the diarrhoea is not appropriate, for example if the diarrhoea, which may not be associated with any form of infection, persists; in these cases antidiarrhoeal drugs are used.

7.2.4.1 Adsorbents

Diarrhoea is often treated with agents such as kaolin, charcoal or methylcellulose. These agents may provide relief by absorbing some of the excess fluid, or, it has been suggested, by absorbing the microbial toxins.

7.2.4.2 Antimotility drugs

Most of the drugs used in relief of diarrhoea act on either the opiate receptors or the muscarinic receptors of the gut. The main opiate drugs used in the treatment of diarrhoea are codeine, diphenoxylate, loperamide and morphine (Box 7.3). All of these drugs have the effect of increasing the tone of the gut but diminishing the peristalsis, they thus relieve the diarrhoea but cause constipation. Morphine and codeine can also cause nausea and vomiting, sedation and drowsiness, etc. (see Chapter 3), due to their actions on the central nervous system; loperamide and diphenoxylate do not cross the blood–brain barrier and are therefore free of such adverse effects.

> Loperamide and diphenoxylate do not cross the blood–brain barrier and therefore do not have the same effects on the central nervous system as morphine

■ *Box 7.3* Antimotility drugs used in the relief of diarrhoea

Drug	*Proprietary name*
Codeine	Diarrest® (liquid)
	Kaodene® (liquid)
Diphenoxylate + atropine	Lomotil® (tablets)
Loperamide	Imodium® (capsules)
Morphine	Kaolin and Morphine (Liquid)

The only antimuscarinic agent used therapeutically for the treatment of diarrhoea is atropine, which is normally co-administered with diphenoxylate.

For many people daily defaecation is seen as a necessity and a virtue

■ **7.2.5 AGENTS USED FOR THE TREATMENT OF CONSTIPATON**

In many cases concern about the lack of gut motility arises from the popular belief that regular 'bowel habits' are a virtue; in some cases, however, the constipation may be a feature of an underlying disorder such as diabetes mellitus or it may be an adverse effect of some other medication.

Constipation can be treated using purgatives, which accelerate the movement of contents through the gut. Purgatives include stimulants, bulking agents and faecal softeners.

7.2.5.1 Stimulant purgatives

These agents increase peristalsis by their direct stimulant actions on the gut. Agents used therapeutically include senna, bisacodyl and sodium picosulphate, which are all known to stimulate the neurones of the myenteric plexus directly. Agents that are available in the form of herbal or 'natural' remedies include phenolphthalein, cascara and juniper berry oil. Stimulant purgatives are widely used by the general public, but their use in conventional therapeutics is limited.

7.2.5.2 Bulking agents

Bulking agents act by increasing the volume of the gut contents and therefore stimulating peristalsis. One form of bulking agent, osmotic laxatives, are essentially solutes which are poorly absorbed from the gut and therefore act to retain fluid within the gut lumen by osmosis. The most commonly used osmotic laxatives are magnesium sulphate and magnesium hydroxide. Another osmotic laxative, lactulose, is a disaccharide which is converted to lactic acid and ethanoic acid by gut bacteria. The products of the conversion act as the osmotic laxatives.

The other form of bulking-forming laxatives are agents such as bran, methylcellulose and stercula. These are not absorbed from the gut but have the effect of retaining fluid, thus increasing the bulk within the gut lumen and stimulating peristalsis.

7.2.5.3 Faecal softeners

Faecal softeners enhance peristalsis by acting as a lubricant and by softening the faeces. Traditional agents include liquid paraffin and arachis oil. Dioctyl sodium sulphosuccinate (docusate sodium) is a surface active agent which also has some stimulant laxative properties; this agent is available for both oral and rectal administration and for use in paediatrics.

■ 7.2.6 DRUGS USED TO ACCELERATE GASTRIC EMPTYING

It is sometime necessary to accelerate gastric emptying time, for example in delayed gastric emptying as a consequence of diabetes mellitus or prior to a surgical procedure. Domperidone and metoclopramide are both antagonists of dopamine D_2 receptors which decrease gastric emptying time and accelerate movement of contents through other areas of the gut. It is unclear whether the clinical effects of these drugs are dependent upon the dopamine antagonism or whether effects at adrenoceptors or muscarinic receptors are more important.

Cisapride acts to increase gut tone and motility by causing the release of acetylcholine within the myenteric plexus.

■ 7.3 DRUGS ACTING ON THE BLADDER

The bladder, like the gut, is comprised of smooth muscle which is not under voluntary control. Bladder contractions occur as a reflex, in response to stimulation of stretch receptors in the bladder; however, the reflex can be suppressed voluntarily. Acetylcholine, acting on muscarinic receptors, causes bladder contraction, thus antimuscarinic agents, such as atropine, are able to prevent these actions of the parasympathetic autonomic nervous system. Such an action explains the urinary retention which is one of the classical anticholinergic side-effects, and explains the fact that some authorities report the (historical) use of anticholinergic agents in incontinent patients to decrease the frequency of micturition.

Anticholinergic agents may have been used historically to facilitate the care of incontinent patients

The only drugs used therapeutically to influence bladder contractions are carbachol and bethanechol, which both act as agonists at the muscarinic receptor and can be used to stimulate bladder emptying in cases of neurological desease or neuronal damage. Drugs such as anticholinesterases (Chapter 2) would have similar actions due to the potentiation of the effects of endogenous acetylcholine.

■ 7.4 DRUGS ACTING ON THE UTERUS
7.4.1 THE PHYSIOLOGY OF THE UTERUS

The uterine smooth muscle differs from other smooth muscles, such as those of the gut and the bladder, because it is influenced directly by reproductive hormones (Chapter 8), and thus its function and activity varies, depending upon the stage of the reproductive (menstrual) cycle or stage of pregnancy. The uterus is comprised of a large body of smooth muscle, the myometrium, lined with cells capable of supporting a developing fetus, the endometrium. The myometrium is innervated by both the sympathetic and the parasympathetics nervous systems, although the sympathetic system predominates. The activity of the endometrium depends upon the endocrine environment, particularly the secretion of oestrogens and progesterone from the ovaries and the secretion of hormones by the feto-placental unit. The effects of hormones on the endometrium are discussed in Chapter 8.

The myometrium is able to contract spontaneously, thus disruption of its nerve supply has little effect. In the non-pregnant uterus there are weak spontaneous contractions, which become stronger towards the latter stages of the menstrual cycle; there is also a burst of uterine activity in the hours following coitus. During early pregnancy the normal uterine contractions are inhibited; contractions re-appear and become stronger and more frequent towards the end of pregnancy. *In vitro*, uterine smooth muscle contracts in response to the posterior pituitary hormone oxytocin, certain prostaglandins, acetylcholine, angiotensin and α-adrenoceptor stimulation; β-adrenoceptor agonists inhibit uterine contractions. Oestrogens and progesterone also tend to inhibit uterine contractions, as

evidenced by the quiescence of the uterus during pregnancy when there are high circulating concentrations of oestrogen and progesterone, but the picture is more complicated than that – fluctuations of oestrogen and progesterone secretion during the normal
menstrual cycle induce variations in the relative expression of α- and β-adrenoceptors,
hence variations in the contractile/inhibitory actions of sympathomimetic agents. Progesterone also inhibits expression of the receptors for oxytocin, this latter effect probably
explains the uterine quiescence during pregnancy; whereas oestrogens increase oxytocin
receptor expression.

Oxytocin, acetylcholine and angiotensin all utilise the same intracellular mechanisms
to induce the contractions. The receptors for all of these agonists are G-protein linked
(Chapter 1), and stimulate the production of inositol triphosphate and diacylglycerol.
The inositol triphosphate is responsible for the liberation of calcium, which ultimately
causes the muscle contraction. Prostaglandins E_2 and $F_{2\alpha}$ cause uterine contractions by
interaction with receptors linked to adenylyl cyclase, thus the second messenger for this
effect is cyclic AMP. Confusingly, the β-adrenergic agonists cause uterine relaxation by
interaction with β_2-adrenoceptors, which also utilise cyclic AMP as the second messenger.
This apparent contradiction can be explained by the concept of discrete intracellular components within the myometrial cells.

■ 7.4.2 UTERINE STIMULANTS AND THEIR USES

There are three clinical situations in which uterine stimulants are of use. The first, and
most common, is the use of stimulants to promote labour when a pregnancy has pro-
gressed beyond full term or when contractions fade during labour. The second is to
induce uterine contractions after the baby has been delivered, this is sometimes done
to reduce or prevent postpartum haemorrhage. The third use of uterine stimulants is to
induce abortion, in this situation the uterine contents are expelled prematurely; the drugs
may also be used to facilitate removal of the uterine contents after miscarriage.

*Uterine stimulants are
used to induce abortion
or to induce labour*

The most potent uterine stimulant is oxytocin, which is prepared synthetically for
therapeutic use. As stated above, oxytocin acts on G-protein coupled receptors to induce powerful uterine contractions, although the number of oxytocin receptors varies,
depending upon the relative concentrations of oestrogens and progesterone. Oxytocin
is therefore most effective at the end of pregnancy when progesterone concentrations
decline. Because of its peptide structure, oxytocin is not orally active and has a short
plasma half-life, because of this it is usually given by intravenous infusion, although the
intramuscular route can also be used. When used to augment labour, oxytocin increases
both the amplitude and the frequency of the uterine contractions, and in excessive doses
can induce a sustained (tetanic) contraction.

Because of its chemical similarity to vasopressin (antidiuretic hormone, see Chapter 4), in high doses oxytocin can also induce adverse cardiovascular effects, most notably
fluid retention and tachycardia. It should also be remembered that another normal physiological role of oxytocin is the induction of contractions in the smooth muscle of the
lactating breast, leading to milk 'let down'. Oxytocin is sometimes therefore used in
postpartum, lactating women to increase the supply of milk. In this situation the oxytocin
is given by nasal spray.

Prostaglandins also induce contractions of the pregnant and non-pregnant uterus, via
generation of cyclic AMP. Prostaglandins E_2 and $F_{2\alpha}$ have the effect of not only promoting
contractions of the uterus, but also ripening (softening) and dilating the uterus; these
effects occur within the 24 hours after administration. Prostaglandins are therefore of

■ *Box 7.4* Drugs used to stimulate uterine contractions

Drug	Proprietary name
Oxytocics	
Oxytocin	Syntocinon® (injection)
Prostaglandins	
Carboprost (PGF$_{2\alpha}$)	Hemabate® (injection)
Dinoprostone (PGE$_2$)	Prepidil® (gel)
	Propess® (pessary)
	Prostin E2® (tablet)
Gemeprost (PGE$_1$)	Gemeprost
Ergots	
Ergometrine	Ergometrine (tablets)
Ergometrine + oxytocin	Syntometrine® (injection)

more use than oxytocin in the induction of pregnancy because of the additional effects on the cervix; premature use of oxytocin may damage the fetus because of the increased uterine contractions against an undilated cervix. Unlike oxytocin, prostaglandins also cause uterine contractions in early or mid pregnancy, and can therefore be used as abortifacients.

Because of their widespread effects elsewhere in the body, prostaglandins are usually given locally, for example by vaginal/cervical pessary or by direct instillation into the amniotic fluid (Box 7.4).

The third group of uterine stimulants are the ergot alkaloids, particularly ergometrine. This agent acts on α-adrenoceptors to induce uterine contractions via synthesis of cyclic AMP, it tends to initiate contractions in quiescent tissues, but has little effect in normally contracting uteri. Its principal clinical uses are for the reduction of blood loss postpartum, or the prevention of blood loss during uterine surgery (for example terminations of pregnancy). The actions of ergometrine on α-adrenoceptors as well as effects on dopamine D$_2$ receptors mean that there are cardiovascular consequences of its use, for example hypertension, and the dopaminergic effects cause nausea and vomiting due to effects on the chemosensory trigger zone (see Section 7.2.3).

■ 7.4.3 UTERINE RELAXANTS AND THEIR USES

Uterine relaxants are used to inhibit uterine contractions when they occur inappropriately early in pregnancy; premature birth is the major cause of infant mortality. Relaxants can also be used in non-pregnant women to relieve the symptoms of dysmenorrhoea. Drugs used to postpone the onset of labour are known as tocolytic agents, of which there are three main types: β-adrenergic agonists, inhibitors of prostaglandin synthesis and competitors for the calcium ion channel.

Drugs used to postpone labour are called tocolytic agents

Selective β$_2$-adrenoceptor agonists such as ritodrine, salbutamol and terbutaline, given by intravenous infusion, can be used to delay the onset of labour for up to 48 hours, although their beneficial effects remain to be fully proven. Because of the ubiquity of β$_2$-adrenoceptors, use of these agents is associated with adverse cardiovascular effects, such as hypotension and tachycardia; the uterine relaxation can also increase blood loss from uterine haemorrhage.

Inhibitors of prostaglandin synthesis, for example non-steroidal anti-inflammatory agents, also reduce uterine contractions, and some workers have shown that these agents are able to delay the onset of labour. They are no longer used for this indication, however, because of adverse effects on the fetus. Inhibitors of prostaglandin synthesis are still used to relax the uterus in non-pregnant women, for example in dysmenorrhoea. Their effectiveness in the relief of this condition is potentiated by their analgesic action, but their use is sometimes questioned because of their inhibitory effects on platelet aggregation and the possibility of increased menstrual blood loss.

Calcium channel blockers, such as those used in the treatment of hypertension, have also been shown to induce uterine relaxation, but as yet they have not been used clinically for this purpose. Another antagonist of the calcium channel, magnesium sulphate, also inhibits uterine motility and can be used as a tocolytic when given by infusion, although its use has been questioned in terms of proven efficacy and potential adverse effects.

■ SUMMARY

- The gastrointestinal tract, bladder and uterus are all smooth-muscle organs. The function of the gut is the digestion of food and the excretion of waste, thus gut dysfunction results in damage of the gut itself due to exposure to digestive forces (ulceration); accelerated excretion of waste and poor digestion (vomiting and diarrhoea) or decreased waste excretion (constipation).

- Drugs used to treat gastric and duodenal ulcers decrease the secretion of gastric acid by antagonism of histamine (H_2) or muscarinic receptors or by inhibition of the proton pump. Another form of treatment, antacids, decreases the deleterious effects of the gastric acid by neutralisation. The drugs used to control vomiting act by antagonism of mucarinic, histamine (H_1), dopamine (D_2) or 5-HT$_3$ receptors of the chemosensory trigger zone (CTZ) of the brain. Drugs used in the treatment of diarrhoea inhibit gut motility either by antagonism of muscarinic receptors or by stimulation of opioid receptors. Some medicines relieve diarrhoea by absorption of fluids and/or toxins. Constipation is treated either by direct irritation of the gut mucosa to cause accelerated peristalsis, increasing the volume of gut contents by use of osmotic laxatives or softening of the faeces.

- Very few drugs are used therapeutically for their actions on the bladder, the exception being muscarinic agonists, which can be used to induce bladder contraction. Anticholinergic agents inhibit bladder contraction and thus cause urinary retention.

- The contractile properties of the uterus varies, depending upon the stage of the menstrual cycle or the stage of pregnancy. Oxytocin is most effective at the end of pregnancy and can be used during labour to promote the normal contractions. Prostaglandins not only cause uterine contractions at any stage of the menstrual cycle or pregnancy, but they also cause softening of the cervix. These agents can therefore be used to induce labour at the end of pregnancy, or to induce premature contractions for the removal of uterine contents following miscarriage or for the purpose of termination of pregnancy. The contractile effects of prostaglandins are also partly responsible for the symptoms of dysmenorrhoea. Ergometrine is most effective in inducing contractions in a quiescent uterus, it is therefore used postpartum to limit uterine haemorrhage. β_2-Adrenoceptor agonists inhibit uterine contractions and can therefore be used to postpone the onset of labour.

■ REVISION QUESTIONS

For each question select the most appropriate answer. Correct answers are presented in Appendix 1.

1. The most important mediator in the secretion of gastric acid is:
   (a) gastrin;
   (b) acetylcholine;
   (c) histamine;
   (d) carbonic anhydrase;
   (e) sodium hydrogen carbonate.

2. The antiemetic agents most effective against the nausea and vomiting induced by anticancer drugs are:
   (a) antimuscarinic agents;
   (b) antagonist of histamine (H_1) receptors;
   (c) antagonists of β_2-adrenoceptors;
   (d) antagonists of 5-HT_3 receptors;
   (e) antagonists of dopamine (D_2) receptors.

3. In a normal, healthy adult the treatment of choice for acute diarrhoea is:
   (a) an antimuscarinic agent;
   (b) loperamide;
   (c) fluid replacement;
   (d) lactulose;
   (e) methylcellulose.

4. Which of the following would *not* be used for the treatment of constipation:
   (a) liquid paraffin;
   (b) methylcellulose;
   (c) sodium picosulphate;
   (d) atropine;
   (e) bisocodyl.

5. When used to promote uterine contractions, oxytocin is given by intravenous infusion because:
   (a) it must be given rapidly;
   (b) it must be given slowly;
   (c) it is not water soluble;
   (d) it is not absorbed from the gastrointestinal tract;
   (e) it causes contractions of the gastrointestinal tract.

6. Agonists of which type of adrenoceptors can be used therapeutically to postpone the onset of labour:
   (a) α_1;
   (b) α_2;
   (c) β_1;
   (d) β_2;
   (e) β_3.

■ SELECTED READING

Burkes, T.F. (1998) Gastrointestinal drugs. In Brody, T.M., Larner, J. and Minneman, K.P. (eds) *Human Pharmacology: Molecular to Clinical* (Third edition), (St. Louis: Mosby), 827–842.

Galbraith, A., Bullock, S., Manias, E., Hunt, B. and Richards, A. (1999) Drugs and the upper gastrointestinal tract. In Galbraith, A., Bullock, S., Manias, E., Hunt, B. and Richards, A. *Fundamentals of Pharmacology*, (Harlow: Addison Wesley Longman), 479–492.

Gard, P.R. (1998) Hormonal control of the gastrointestinal tract. In Gard, P.R. *Modules in Life Science: Human endocrinology*, (London: Taylor & Francis), 69–83.

Mitchell, B.F. (1998) Drugs affecting uterine motility. In Brody, T.M., Larner, J. and Minneman, K.P. (eds) *Human Pharmacology: Molecular to Clinical* (Third edition), (St. Louis: Mosby), 559–571.

Rang, H.P., Dale, M.M. and Ritter, J.M. (1995) The gastrointestinal system. In Rang, H.P., Dale, M.M. and Ritter, J.M. *Pharmacology* (Fourth edition), (Edinburgh: Churchill Livingstone), 370–384.

■ COMPUTER-AIDED LEARNING PACKAGE

Further details of this learning package can be found at
http://www.coacs.com/PCCAL/

Diseases of the Gastrointestinal Tract (Constipation, Diarrhoea and Indigestion) (version 3.0), Pharmacy Consortium for Computer Aided Learning (PCCAL), COACS Ltd, University of Bath.

PHARMACOLOGICAL MANIPULATION OF THE ENDOCRINE SYSTEM

■ 8.1 INTRODUCTION

The endocrine system complements the nervous system in controlling functions such as metabolism, growth and reproduction. It is a major system, comprised of eight major glands. The first is the hypothalamus, which is part of the brain; it is at the level of the hypothalamus that the endocrine system and the central nervous system are co-ordinated. The next gland in the hierarchy of the endocrine system is the pituitary gland. This gland, situated at the base of the skull, behind the eyes, is divided into two independent portions. The anterior portion of the pituitary gland is a development of the brain and receives hormonal signals from the hypothalamus to control its activity; it secretes the trophic hormones, namely thyroid stimulating hormone, adrenocorticotrophic hormone, follicle stimulating hormone and luteinizing hormone, which control the actions of the thyroid gland, adrenal cortex and gonads, respectively. The anterior pituitary gland also secretes growth hormone, which controls growth during childhood and adolescence, and prolactin, which controls milk production by the lactating breast and also has some influence on fertility. The other portion of the pituitary gland is the posterior pituitary, this secretes antidiuretic hormone, which acts on the kidneys to regulate water excretion and fluid balance, and oxytocin, which stimulates milk ejection from the lactating breast and uterine contraction, particularly during parturition.

The thyroid gland is responsible for the regulation of metabolic rate, and is integrally concerned in the process of maturation during childhood. The thyroid gland, together with the parathyroid glands, also controls calcium balance by influencing calcium absorption and excretion and bone formation and breakdown.

The hormones of the pancreas, insulin and glucagon, together with the glucocorticoids from the adrenal cortex, regulate carbohydrate metabolism. The glucocorticoids are also involved in the body's response to stress, as are the hormones of the adrenal medulla. Aldosterone, another hormone secreted by the adrenal cortex, is concerned with sodium balance, and indirectly, fluid balance. The sex hormones from the ovaries and testes are responsible for the development of female and male secondary sexual characteristics, respectively, and play a major role in the initiation and maintenance of fertility.

Most disorders of the endocrine glands stem from either an under-secretion of a hormone, or an over-secretion. In the case of the former the usual approach to treatment is simple hormone replacement therapy (Box 8.1). This is effective in most cases, although

Many disorders of the endocrine glands stem from an over-secretion of a hormone; one form of treatment is the use of hormone receptor antagonists to reduce the effects of this excessive hormone secretion

■ *Box 8.1* Some available preparations for use in hormone replacement therapy

	Hormone	**Proprietary name**
Thyroid gland		
	Thyroxine	Eltroxin® (tablets)
	Tri-iodothyronine	Tertroxin® (tablets)
	Calcitonin (salmon)	Calsynar® (injection)
		Miacalcic® (injection)
Pancreas		
	Insulin (human)	Human Actrapid® (injection)
		Humulin S® (injection)
	Insulin (bovine)	Hypurin® Bovine Neutral (injection)
Adrenal cortex		
	Fludrocortisone	Florinef® (tablets)
	Hydrocortisone	Hydrocortone® (tablets)
Ovaries		
	Oestradiol	Climaval® (tablets)
	Oestradiol	Fematrix® (patches)
	Progesterone	
Testes		
	Testosterone	

it has often proved necessary to develop analogues of the natural hormone with reduced first-pass metabolism, prolonged plasma half-life, etc. Treatment of excessive secretion of hormones is often by surgical removal of all, or part, of the gland in question. Another approach, however, is the use of hormone receptor antagonists to reduce the effects of excessive hormone secretion, or other drugs which reduce synthesis or secretion of the hormone. This chapter will describe the more common endocrine disorders and the drug therapies available, it will also outline the therapeutic uses of hormones.

■ **8.2 THE TREATMENT OF THYROID DISORDERS AND THERAPEUTIC USE OF THYROID HORMONES**

The thyroid gland has two separate functions: first, it secretes calcitonin, which is involved in the control of calcium balance; and, secondly, it secretes tri-iodothyronine and tetra-iodothyronine (sometimes called thyroxine), which are concerned with growth and metabolism. Disorders of calcium balance are discussed in Section 8.3, this section will only cover the treatment of disorders in the secretion of tri-iodothyronine and tetra-iodothyronine, collectively called the thyroid hormones.

■ **8.2.1 HYPOTHYROIDISM**

In adults, undersecretion of thyroid hormones results in decreased basal metabolic rate, the predominant features of which are decreased heart rate with decreased respiration rate and body temperature. There may also be some weight gain due to the decreased utilisation of carbohydrate and fat stores, and decreased neuronal function resulting in slowed reflexes, feelings of tiredness and lethargy and possible psychological disorders such as depression. The condition often causes dry, flaky skin with hair loss and oedema; this oedema resulted in the condition being named myxoedema. Because of the disruption of other endocrine glands, symptoms of hypothyroidism may also include menorrhagia (irregular menstruation) in females and reduced fertility in both males and females.

If the condition occurs prior to adulthood, hypothyroidism causes delayed puberty coupled with diminished linear growth. Hypothyroidism that occurs *in utero*, or in the neonate, carries the risk of severe mental retardation, short stature with oedema and a protruding tongue, which give rise to coarse features and a hoarse cry. This is the condition known as cretinism.

The treatment of thyroid hypoactivity is relatively straightforward if the condition is due to hormonal hyposecretion. The most common form of treatment is hormone replacement therapy with oral tetra-iodothyronine (thyroxine). Tetra-iodothyronine is favoured over tri-iodothyronine firstly on the grounds of cost and, secondly, because of its longer plasma half-life. Administration of excessive replacement doses may cause cardiovascular problems and other symptoms of hyperthyroidism (see Section 8.2.2).

One possible cause of hypothyroidism is iodine deficiency, in such patients oral iodine supplemention is effective, although administration of excessive doses of iodine paradoxically results in further decreases in thyroid hormone synthesis.

> The treatment of thyroid hypoactivity is relatively straightforward if the condition is due to hormonal hyposecretion. The most common form of treatment for thyroid hypoactivity is replacement therapy with thyroxine

■ 8.2.2 HYPERTHYROIDISM

The symptoms of hyperthyroidism are those of increased metabolism, such as tachycardia and possible cardiac arrhythmias, excessive sweating, agitation, anxiety and weight loss despite increased appetite. Osteoporosis and amenorrhoea may also occur, and in nearly all cases there is a goitre (Section 8.2.3). The most common cause of hyperthyroidism is Graves' disease, which is characterised by exophthalmos (bulging eyes).

The drug treatment of Graves' disease and other forms of hyperthyroidism involves the use of anti-thyroid drugs, although many of the symptoms of hyperthyroidism can be relieved by use of β-adrenoceptor antagonists (Chapter 2). Exophthalmos is sometimes treated with immunosuppressant doses of corticosteroids (Section 8.5).

> The drug treatment of Graves' disease involves the inhibition of thyroid hormone synthesis

The anti-thyroid drug carbimazole acts by inhibition of the synthesis of thyroid hormones by preventing the incorporation of the iodine moiety into the thyroid hormone molecule. Potassium perchlorate acts in a similar way by competing with iodide for uptake into the thyroid gland. The drug therapy is usually continued for 12 to 24 months. Careful selection of the dose allows normal thyroid hormone concentrations to be achieved, but remission occurs in about half of the patients when drug therapy is stopped. Neo-Mercazole® (carbimazole) is a preparation currently available in the UK.

■ 8.2.3 GOITRE

Goitre is an enlargement of the thyroid gland which is manifested as a swelling of the neck. Goitre may be a symptom of either an over-active or under-active thyroid gland, and is therefore usually resolved upon appropriate treatment of the underlying thyroid disorder. However, some drugs can induce goitre. Lithium, which is used in the treatment of manic depression (Chapter 3), may cause goitre, as may certain iodides which are contained in vitamin preparations and some cough remedies.

> Iodides contained in vitamin preparations and some cough remedies may cause goitre

■ 8.3 DISORDERS OF THE ENDOCRINE CONTROL OF CALCIUM BALANCE AND THEIR TREATMENT

The hormones that are normally involved in the control of calcium balance are parathyroid hormone (PTH) from the parathyroid gland; calcitonin, which is secreted by the thyroid gland; and 1,25-dihydroxycholecalciferol (1,25-DHCC), which is produced in the kidneys. Calcitonin has the effect of decreasing plasma calcium concentrations by decreasing its liberation from bone and increasing its excretion; parathyroid hormone and 1,25-DHCC increase plasma calcium concentrations by a combination of increased calcium absorption by the gut, increased calcium liberation from bone, decreased bone formation and decreased calcium excretion. The three hormones act together to maintain appropriate bone turnover and to keep plasma calcium concentrations within the normal physiological range.

■ 8.3.1 HYPOPARATHYROIDISM

Removal of the parathyroid glands results in death within hours; however, a relative deficiency of PTH is often symptomless, or may be limited to paraesthesia of the fingers and toes. Long-term hypoparathyroidism may result in tetany, convulsions and cataracts. The major biochemical feature of hypoparathyroidism is low plasma calcium (hypocalcaemia), thus its treatment is by calcium supplementation together with replacement therapy, with either parathyroid hormone, which is expensive, or an analogue of 1,25-DHCC such as vitamin D.

■ 8.3.2 HYPERPARATHYROIDISM

Hyperparathyroidism,
which may result in
muscle weakness,
cardiac arrhythmias
and mental confusion,
can be treated with
biphosphonates

Hyperparathyroidism is usually diagnosed after a long period of illness, during investigations of other conditions. Its predominant symptoms are those caused by the increased plasma calcium (hypercalcaemia); thus there is tiredness, lethargy and a general feeling of being unwell, there may also be polyuria with dehydration. If untreated, the condition may progress with an increase in muscle weakness, cardiac arrhythmias and mental confusion. The condition may ultimately result in coma or death.

Drug treatment of hyperparathyroidism involves the use of drugs such as the diuretic frusemide, to potentiate excretion of calcium; the administration of one of a group of drugs called biphosphonates, which directly inhibit bone resorption; or the administration of salmon calcitonin, to counteract the effects of the parathyroid hormone.

■ 8.4 DISORDERS OF THE ENDOCRINE PANCREAS AND THEIR TREATMENT

Many hormones affect carbohydrate metabolism, but the most important are the pancreatic hormones insulin and glucagon. Insulin acts to decrease plasma glucose concentrations by increasing its utilisation and storage and by decreasing its formation. Glucagon, on the other hand, increases plasma glucose concentrations by promoting the liberation of glucose from glycogen and fat stores. The secretion of insulin following food intake and the secretion of glucagon during fasting results in the maintenance of stable plasma glucose concentrations.

■ 8.4.1 DIABETES MELLITUS

Deficiency of insulin results in the inability of tissues to take up and utilise glucose, and the inability to store glucose. The symptoms of the associated condition are therefore weight loss, tiredness and lethargy, and diminished growth; this condition is called insulin dependent diabetes mellitus (IDDM), and it usually develops in children. The presenting symptoms of IDDM are usually excessive urine output and excessive thirst, due to glucose excretion, but if left untreated, the starvation of tissues that occurs in IDDM can result in blindness, peripheral vascular disease, peripheral neuropathy and ultimately death.

If left untreated, diabetes
mellitus can cause
blindness, peripheral
vascular disease,
peripheral neuropathy
and ultimately death

As the name suggests, the treatment of IDDM is dependent upon insulin replacement; to date there is no other form of medication that is able to overcome the pancreatic deficit. The earliest form of insulin to be used therapeutically was obtained from the pancreases

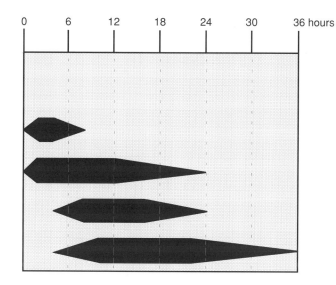

Preparation

Neutral Insulin

Biphasic Insulin

Insulin Zinc Suspension

Protamine Zinc Insulin

• **Figure 8.1** A representation of the different formulations of insulin, their speeds of onset and duration of action. ◄, Time to onset of action; ■, peak action; ►, time to offset of action

of cows or pigs. These bovine and porcine insulins are active in humans despite the fact that they differ from human insulin in one or three amino acids, respectively. Modern therapeutics has switched to replacement therapy using human insulin, which has the advantage that it is not recognised as a foreign protein and therefore does not precipitate antibody formation. This human insulin is made either by the enzymatic conversion of porcine insulin, or by biotechnological procedures using either *Escherichia coli* or yeast (*Saccharomyces cerevisiae*).

Because insulin is a peptide, it cannot be administered orally (Chapter 10). The most common form of administration is therefore by injection; the usual sites of injection being the upper arms, thighs, lower abdomen or the buttocks. Once injected, the insulin undergoes distribution within the blood to the target tissues before it is degraded, predominantly by the liver. Following subcutaneous or intramuscular administration, insulin can be detected in the blood for up to 3 hours. Different formulations of insulin have been developed to vary the duration of action of the injected insulin (figure 8.1), for example the injection of a simple solution of insulin may be sufficient to lower blood glucose for a period of 1–4 hours. Injection of long-acting insulin, developed by the addition of either zinc or protamine to the insulin solution, can lower blood glucose for up to 24 hours. In practice, most diabetics are treated with a combination of a short-acting and a long-acting insulin. During insulin therapy food intake must be matched to the administered dose of insulin. Insufficient intake of carbohydrate results in hypoglycaemia, the symptoms of which are lethargy, dizziness and confusion; whereas excessive carbohydrate intake results in hyperglycaemia. The dose of insulin and the diet must also be matched to the predicted physical activity to be undertaken, thus a sedentary office worker requires a lower food intake and insulin dose than a manual labourer.

Another form of diabetes mellitus is non-insulin dependent diabetes mellitus (NIDDM). This condition arises because the secreted insulin is unable to produce an effect, commonly due to defective insulin receptors. Patients with NIDDM are usually about 50 years old and overweight; the excessive weight is probably responsible for the condition. The symptoms and consequences of NIDDM are similar to those of IDDM except that IDDM patients are usually thin and wasting. In NIDDM it is believed that the excessive storage of fat results in damage to the membrane-bound, tyrosine-kinase-linked

• **Figure 8.2** The mechanism of action of sulphonylurea oral hypoglycaemic drugs

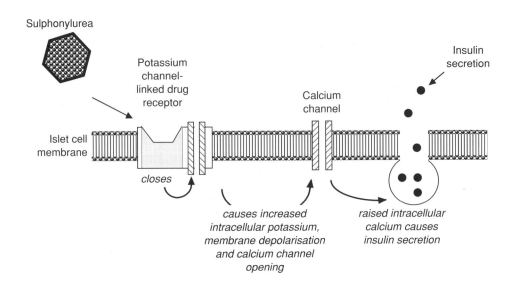

insulin receptor; the first line of treatment of NIDDM is therefore dietary control aimed at weight loss. In many cases the depletion of fat stores and the resultant weight loss is sufficient to relieve the NIDDM, but in those in whom dietary control is ineffective an alternative therapy is necessary.

Oral hypoglycaemic agents are drugs which, when taken orally, confer some control over carbohydrate metabolism. Their use is limited by the fact that they appear to re-quire a functioning pancreas in order to produce their effect, thus they can only be used in the treatment of NIDDM, not IDDM. In the treatment of NIDDM, these drugs have their greatest effect on basal blood glucose concentration; they have little effect on the raised blood glucose that occurs after food intake, thus their use is usually coupled with dietary control.

The most commonly used group of oral hypoglycaemic agents are the sulphonylurea drugs such as chlorpropamide, glibenclamide, tolbutamide and glipizide. These drugs bind to the surface of the β-cells of the islets of Langerhans to stimulate insulin secre-tion. They appear to do this by interacting with specific membrane-bound receptors, resulting in a decrease in potassium efflux, partial depolarisation of the cell membrane and influx of calcium ions. It is this calcium influx which causes the secretion of insulin (figure 8.2). These drugs also sensitise the β-cells to stimuli that cause insulin secretion, possibly by raising intracellular levels of the second messenger cAMP as a consequence of inhibition of phosphodiesterase. In high concentrations, sulphonylureas also increase insulin-mediated tissue uptake of glucose and increase insulin receptor density, although these actions are probably irrelevant at therapeutic doses. These drugs are effective in the treatment of many cases of NIDDM, but they are not without side-effects, one of which is that they tend to produce an increase in weight, in a population being treated for a disorder which may be a consequence of obesity.

Another group of oral hypoglycaemic agents is the biguanide drugs, of which the only one available for clinical use is metformin. This drug acts by enhancing peripheral uptake of glucose and by reducing gluconeogenesis. It is an effective drug, but its usefulness is limited by the fact that it sometimes causes profound lactic acidaemia, which may be fatal.

Oral hypoglycaemic agents are drugs which are limited by the fact that they require a functioning pancreas to produce their effect

■ 8.5 DISORDERS OF THE ADRENAL GLAND AND THE USE OF ADRENAL HORMONES AND THEIR ANALOGUES

The adrenal gland is comprised of two separate components, the inner adrenal medulla, which secretes adrenaline and noradrenaline, and the outer adrenal cortex, which secretes adrenocortical hormones. There are many different adrenocortical hormones but they can be grouped into three classes: the glucocorticoids, the mineralocorticoids and the androgens. Androgens are discussed in Section 8.6.

■ 8.5.1 THE ADRENAL MEDULLA

The adrenal medulla secretes adrenaline and noradrenaline at times of stress. These two catecholamines have similar actions via their effects on α- and β-adrenoceptors (Chapter 1), although noradrenaline acts predominantly on α-adrenoceptors whereas adrenaline has a greater effect on β-adrenoceptors. The overall effect of the hormones of the adrenal medulla is often referred to as the 'fight or flight' response, as they produce an increase in heart and respiration rate, increased blood flow to muscles, increased blood glucose and increased mental alertness. The therapeutic uses of adrenaline, noradrenaline and their analogues (sympathomimetics) are discussed in Chapter 2.

The most important disorder of the adrenal medulla is phaeochromocytoma, a tumour that causes increased, but often sporadic, secretion of adrenaline and noradrenaline. Typical symptoms are short-lived attacks of panic, sweating, pallor, chest pain and severe headache, which may be precipitated by factors such as emotion, exercise or some foodstuffs. There may also be postural hypotension, although there are also cases of hypertension. Short-term control of the symptoms of phaeochromocytoma may be achieved by use of pharmacological antagonists for α- and β-adrenoceptors (Chapter 2).

■ 8.5.2 THE ADRENAL CORTEX

All of the hormones of the adrenal cortex share a similar chemical structure, based upon a cyclopentenoperhydrophenanthrene ring structure (figure 8.3). Hormones with similar structures are also secreted by the ovaries and the testes. These are the steroid hormones, and drugs developed from them are usually collectively called steroids.

Hormones from the adrenal cortex, and drugs developed from them, are usually collectively called steroids

The two major groups of hormones which are secreted by the adrenal cortex are the glucocorticoids and the mineralocorticoids. Glucocorticoids are released at times of stress and they have the effect of increasing plasma glucose concentrations, decreasing the extent of any inflammation at sites of tissue damage, suppressing the immune system and producing psychological effects such as euphoria and sedation. All of these effects are aimed at allowing the individual to perform despite the presence of stress or injury. The

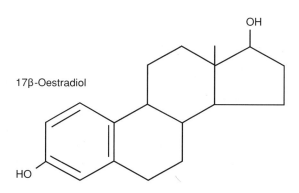

17β-Oestradiol

• **Figure 8.3** The chemical structure of a typical steroid hormone, in this case 17β-oestradiol

secretion of glucocorticoids is stimulated by adrenocorticotrophic hormone (ACTH) from the anterior pituitary gland and corticotrophin releasing hormone (CRH) from the hypothalamus. The secretion of glucocorticoids, the most important of which is cortisol, is under negative feedback control by the hypothalamus and the anterior pituitary gland.

The most important mineralocorticoid is aldosterone; although chemically similar to cortisol, and secreted by the same endocrine gland, the secretion of aldosterone is independent of cortisol secretion, being controlled by the activity of the renin–angiotensin system (Chapter 4). Aldosterone causes increased sodium reabsorption by the kidney, with increased potassium excretion, which in turn increases blood osmolarity, blood volume and blood pressure.

8.5.2.1 Disorders of mineralocorticoid secretion

A deficiency of mineralocorticoids results in excessive excretion of sodium, which may produce hypotension, although in most cases other compensatory mechanisms are able to maintain the blood pressure within the normal physiological range. Where symptoms do arise, however, they can be controlled by administration of drugs such as fludrocortisone, which mimic the actions of aldosterone.

Excess secretion of mineralocorticoids results in hypertension, because of the sodium and fluid retention, coupled with hypokalaemia which induces muscle weakness. The usual form of treatment for hyperaldosteronism (Conn's syndrome) is the surgical removal of the tumour, although in some cases the condition can be controlled by use of the aldosterone receptor antagonist spironolactone, which prevents the actions of aldosterone at its receptor.

Excessive secretion of mineralocorticoids results in hypertension and muscle weakness, but can be controlled using an aldosterone receptor antagonist

8.5.2.2 Disorders of glucocorticoid secretion

Decreased secretion of glucocorticoids may be due to a disease of the adrenal cortex itself, or a disorder of the secretion of ACTH or CRF by the anterior pituitary or hypothalamus, respectively. The lack of glucocorticoid secretion (Addison's disease) causes hypoglycaemia and thus symptoms of tiredness and weakness. In the rare cases where the onset of the disease is rapid, the presenting symptoms may be hypotension, nausea, vomiting, diarrhoea, confusion and coma, which may culminate in death within 24 hours. If the disease is slower in onset, there may be a single symptom of tiredness or a more extensive condition with tiredness, weakness, anorexia and weight loss. Prolonged deficiency of glucocorticoids may be accompanied by an increase in the secretion of ACTH due to the release of the anterior pituitary gland from negative feedback; increased ACTH produces skin pigmentation reminiscent of a sun tan. Treatment of the glucocorticoid deficiency is by administration of a glucocorticoid such as hydrocortisone or, more rarely, by administration of an ACTH analogue.

Treatment of Addison's disease is by administration of a glucocorticoid such as hydrocortisone or, more rarely, by administration of an ACTH analogue

Increased secretion of glucocorticoids is referred to as Cushing's syndrome. Again, the condition may arise because of a disorder of the adrenal cortex, or it may involve overactivity of the hypothalamus or anterior pituitary gland. Cushing's syndrome may also develop following excessive intake of steroid drugs (Section 8.5.2.3). The symptoms of Cushing's syndrome reflect the multiple actions of the glucocorticoids: thus there is hyperglycaemia, resulting in polyuria and polydipsia, and a loss of muscle mass due to increased protein metabolism. Other actions of the glucocorticoids also become apparent at these high circulating concentrations, thus mineralocorticoid-like effects of glucocorticoids induce sodium and fluid retention, resulting in hypertension, and androgenic effects cause acne and excessive hair growth with menstrual disturbances in women (Section

8.7). If left untreated, Cushing's syndrome usually proves fatal within 5 years, death being due to cardiovascular disease, complications of diabetes mellitus or infection.

The usual treatment of Cushing's syndrome is the surgical removal of the tumour, although destruction of the affected gland is sometimes achieved using external irradiation. Drugs are available to inhibit the normal synthesis of the adrenal steroids by inhibition of either 11β-hydroxylase or 3β-hydroxysteroid dehydrogenase, but these usually only provide temporary relief because of an increased secretion of ACTH; there are no pharmacological antagonists of glucocorticoid receptors.

Cushing's disease is caused by excess glucocorticoid activity; there are no pharmacological antagonists of glucocorticoid receptors

8.5.2.3 Pharmacological uses of adrenocorticosteroids

Mineralocorticoids are used only for replacement therapy (Section 8.5.2.1); however, because of its short plasma half-life, aldosterone is unsuitable, the drug of choice is thus fludrocortisone.

Glucocorticoids are used in replacement therapy for the treatment of conditions such as Addison's disease, for their immunosuppressive or anti-inflammatory effects in the treatment of conditions such as arthritis, asthma or allergies, or for the treament of proliferative conditions such as leukaemia. In most cases, the selection of the glucocorticoid is dependent upon the pharmacokinetics of the available agents and the predominant effect required; most glucocorticoids are orally active but their absorption through the skin varies, as does their plasma half-life. For replacement therapy, the natural hormones cortisol and cortisone, which must undergo conversion to cortisol, are the drugs of choice because they have limited immunosuppressive activity but high mineralocorticoid activity. In the treatment of inflammatory conditions, prednisolone, methylprednisolone and prednisone, which is converted to prednisolone, are of use because they have good anti-inflammatory/immunosuppressant effects with minimal mineralocorticoid actions. Dexamethasone and betamethasone are also very potent immunosuppressants with minimal mineralocorticoid activity, but their long plasma half-life and their growth-suppressing properties render them unsuitable for long-term use; they are therefore only used for the treatment of severe, acute inflammatory disorders (Box 8.2).

Glucocorticoids are used for the treatment of Addison's disease, for their immunosuppressive or anti-inflammatory effects in the treatment of conditions such as arthritis, asthma or allergies, or for the treatment of proliferative conditions such as leukaemia

Many adverse effects are associated with the use of glucocorticoids. The development of diabetes mellitus and other symptoms of Cushing's syndrome may accompany steroid therapy, and there may be suppression of wound healing and exacerbation of infections due to immunosuppressant effects. Long-term use in children may cause inhibition of growth, and in adults may result in osteoporosis. Probably the most important adverse effect, however, is suppression of the hypothalamic–pituitary axis. Chronic administration of exogenous glucocorticoids results in suppression of ACTH secretion which, in turn, leads to atrophy of the adrenal cortex. If steroid therapy is then stopped abruptly, the adrenal cortex is unable to secrete endogenous hormones and the patient suffers an Addisonian crisis, which may be fatal. It is this phenomenon which has given rise to the public perception that it is possible to become 'addicted' to steroid drugs; steroids are not addictive in the true pharmacological sense. These consequences of cessation of steroid therapy are overcome by the gradual reduction of the dose of the exogenous steroid, in order to allow regeneration of the adrenal gland. Other consequences of suppression of the anterior pituitary may include disturbances of sex hormone secretion, resulting in symptoms such as menstrual disturbances (Section 8.7). It should always be remembered that the use of corticosteroids for suppression of the inflammatory response has the effect of removing the symptoms without affecting the cause of the underlying disorder, which may worsen.

There are many adverse effects of steroid therapy

■ *Box 8.2* Currently available drugs which are based on adrenal steroids (reproduced from Gard, P.R. (1998) *Modules in Life Science: Human endocrinology*, London: Taylor & Francis)

Corticosteroids are used widely to control the symptoms of a variety of disorders which involve an inflammatory or an immune response. These drugs may be used either systemically (in the form of tablets or injections) or locally (in the form of creams, inhalers or nasal sprays). All of the corticosteroids used are potent glucocorticoids with little or no mineralocorticoid or androgenic actions.

Drug	Relative potency*	Proprietary name
Hydrocortisone	1	Efcortelan® (cream), Canesten HC® (cream), Daktacort® (cream)
Prednisolone	5	Precortisyl Forte® (tablets), Prednesol® (tablets)
Methylprednisolone	6	Medrone® (tablets, injections)
Triamcinolone	6	Kenalog® (injection)
Betamethasone	30	Betnelan® (tablets), Betnovate® (cream), Betnesol® (tablets, injection, drops)
Dexamethasone	30	Decadron® (tablets, injection)
Beclomethasone (beclometasone)	125	AeroBec® (inhaler), Becotide® (inhaler), Beconase® (nasal spray), Propaderm® (cream)
Budesonide	125	Pulmicort® (inhaler), Rhinocort® (nasal spray)
Fluticasone	250	Flixotide® (inhaler), Flixonase® (nasal spray)
Flunisolide	250	Syntaris® (nasal spray)

* Approximate potency, higher values represent greater potency. No account is taken of the duration of action.

■ 8.6 THERAPEUTIC USES OF MALE SEX HORMONES AND THE PHARMACOLOGICAL TREATMENT OF MALE REPRODUCTIVE DISORDERS

Male sex hormones or androgens, the most important of which is testosterone, are secreted predominantly by the testes, although there is also some secretion by the ovaries and the adrenal cortex. Under normal circumstances only those male sex hormones secreted by the testes are of physiological significance. Like the glucorticoids, the male sex hormones all share a chemical structure based upon the cyclopentenoperhydrophenanthrene nucleus; the hormones and related drugs are therefore usually known collectively as the androgenic steroids.

The physiological effects of the androgens are concerned with development of male anatomy, thus *in utero* they induce development of male genitalia, and at puberty they cause development of male secondary sexual characteristics such as facial hair, muscle development, long bone growth and psychological changes such as aggressiveness and increased libido. Androgens, in combination with follicle stimulating hormone (FSH) from the anterior pituitary gland, are also necessary for sperm production.

In those genetic males in whom there is a lack of androgen secretion or an inability to respond to testosterone *in utero*, there is a failure to develop male genitalia; the infant is therefore born with either female or ambiguous genitalia. If the androgen deficiency occurs after birth but before puberty, there will be a lack of, or a delay in, the development of the male secondary sexual chartacteristics. The features of this condition are described as eunuchoid because there is no increase in muscle mass, enlargement of the larynx or growth of pubic hair, the external genitalia also remain infantile and there is no sperm production. If the deficiency occurs after puberty, there is a decrease or cessation of sperm production with loss of muscle mass and pubic hair. There is also a decrease in libido and aggression; there is little or no change in voice. Treatment of these conditions may necessitate androgen replacement therapy, or if fertility and sperm production are required, administration of gonadotrophins (Sections 8.6.1 and 8.8, and Box 8.3).

Excessive testosterone in an adult male normally goes unrecognized because of the wide variation in the extent of androgen activity seen in the normal population. Such conditions can occur, however, in cases of testicular or adrenal tumours or in individuals misusing therapeutic androgens for their anabolic actions (Section 8.6.1). The usual presenting symptom would be that of decreased fertility, possible with some testicular atrophy. These symptoms arise because of the suppression of gonadotrophin secretion by the anterior pituitary. Excessive or inappropriate secretion of androgens in young males may produce precocious puberty – onset of puberty before the age of 9 is considered abnormal. Androgen-secreting tumours may also occur in females. The effects of the androgens in females would be to cause enlargement of the clitoris with development of male-pattern pubic hair (including facial hair) and an increase in muscle mass. There would also be a deepening of the voice and excessive activity of the sebaceous glands; there may also be increases in libido and aggression. The actions of the androgens on the anterior pituitary gland would cause disruption of the menstrual cycle. If the condition remains untreated, it may result in baldness. Precocious puberty in juvenile males and masculinisation in females may be treated by administration of an androgen receptor antagonist such as cyproterone acetate, or by removal of the source of the hormone. Cyproterone acetate has also been used for the control of excessive aggression and/or libido in adult males where the underlying cause may be excessive secretion of androgens (Section 8.6.2).

Cyproterone acetate has been used for the control of aggression and excessive libido in males

■ 8.6.1 THERAPEUTIC USES OF ANDROGENS

Androgenic steroids may be used for hormone replacement therapy in the treatment of hypogonadism in males, but because of their ability to increase muscle mass, their anabolic actions, they are sometimes used in the treatment of certain wasting disorders. The anabolic androgenic steroids have also been misused by athletes in an attempt to increase muscle mass and strength. There is some evidence of their efficacy; however, it is possible that their actions owe more to their glucocorticoid activity (Section 8.5) than to the anabolic/androgenic actions. It has been suggested that the use of steroids by athletes enables them to continue training for longer, being less affected by fatigue or injury, to attain greater strength and to improve performance because of increased aggression. When used therapeutically, testosterone is usually administered by injection within an oil vehicle, this route of administration avoids the first-pass metabolism by the liver and hence provides sustained androgen activity. Orally active synthetic androgenic/anabolic steroids, such as stanozolol, have also been produced.

Anabolic steroids have been abused by athletes in an attempt to enhance performance

The side-effects of anabolic steroid abuse are predictable. In adult males, the only manifest side-effect is infertility and testicular atrophy due to the suppression of gonadotrophin secretion; in some cases this effect may be irreversible. There may also be increased risks of cardiovascular disease and prostate carcinoma. In adult females, the use of anabolic steroids results in disruption of the menstrual cycle, clitoral enlargement and development of male-pattern pubic hair. If the drugs are used in children, they can cause precocious development of male secondary sexual characteristics in both males and females.

■ 8.6.2 PHARMACOLOGICAL TREATMENT OF EXCESSIVE ANDROGEN ACTIVITY

Excessive stimulation of androgen-responsive tissues by androgenic hormones may result in uncontrolled cellular replication, for example prostate cancer. Prostate cancer is thus an example of a hormone-dependent cancer, and treatment therefore aims to deprive the tumour of the androgens required for its continued growth. This effect can be achieved in several different ways: removal of the source of endogenous hormones; prevention of the synthesis or secretion of the hormones; use of a pharmacological antagonist of the hormones; or use of a physiological antagonist of the hormones.

The removal of the source of the hormones is usually a surgical procedure and therefore beyond the scope of this text. Another method to reduce the secretion of the androgens is to administer an analogue of gonadotrophin releasing hormone (GnRH). GnRH is normally secreted by the hypothalamus and it has the effect of stimulating the anterior pituitary gland to secrete luteinising hormone (LH). LH, in turn, stimulates testosterone secretion from the testes. GnRH analogues mimic the actions of endogenous GnRH and therefore initially stimulate the secretion of LH and ultimately testosterone. After about 10 days of use, however, the GnRH receptors down-regulate, which results in complete inhibition of LH secretion and therefore cessation of testosterone production. As described above, the effects of androgens can also be reduced by the administration of androgen receptor antagonists such as cyproterone acetate. These drugs have the advantage that they also reduce the effects of androgens of adrenal origin, but the disadvantage that they remove the effects of negative feedback, and therefore may induce an increased secretion of LH from the antererior pituitary gland. An alternative approach is to use high-dose oestrogen therapy (Section 8.7); this form of treatment has the effect of reducing the influence of the androgens, by acting in an opposing manner, but carries with it a wide range of adverse effects dependent upon the oestrogenic effects, for example gynaecomastia and an increased risk of thromboembolism.

■ 8.6.3 MALE HORMONAL CONTRACEPTIVES

The aim of a male contraceptive is to suppress sperm production in a reversible manner. As already described, initiation of sperm production is dependent upon the presence of both FSH and testosterone, but once initiated sperm production can, in some individuals, be maintained by testosterone alone. Several regimes have been tested as male contraceptives (Box 8.4). The most obvious is the administration of an androgen receptor antagonist, but this has the effect of reducing sperm count and at the same time causing regression of some of the male secondary sexual characteristics, including a decrease in libido. These side-effects render this form of contraception unusable. Another method has used GnRH analogues, which suppress the secretion of LH and FSH due to down-regulation of the GnRH receptors. There is a marked decrease in sperm production, but the inhibition of LH secretion induces testosterone deficiency, again causing regression of secondary sexual characteristics; the suppression of FSH secretion may also cause testicular atrophy. Some of these problems can be overcome by administration of the drug danazol, which is an inhibitor of LH and FSH secretion but also possesses slight androgenic properties. Other attempts to suppress FSH secretion in males have used the female sex hormone analogue medroxyprogesterone (Section 8.7) in combination with testosterone replacement. There was limited success, but trials were discontinued because of fears of progestogenic and oestrogenic side-effects.

The most successful male hormonal contraceptive has been testosterone enanthate, given by weekly intramuscular injection. This treatment acts by the suppression of LH and FSH secretion, but overcomes the problems of the regimes described above because it has inherent androgen replacement. Contraceptive efficacy comparable with that obtained by female oral contraceptives has been reported, although the treatment was effective in only about 60% of users. There were some reports of side-effects such as weight gain, decreased testicular volume, acne and increased aggression and libido, but the major drawback is patient compliance with the weekly injections.

> The most successful form of male hormonal contraceptive is as effective as female oral contraceptives

■ 8.7 THERAPEUTIC USES OF FEMALE SEX HORMONES AND THE PHARMACOLOGICAL TREATMENT OF FEMALE REPRODUCTIVE DISORDERS

Like the androgens, the female sex hormones also share the basic steroid structure. The predominant female sex hormones are oestradiol and progesterone. Oestradiol is the most important member of a group of related hormones called the oestrogens. These hormones are secreted by the Graafian follicles and, to a lesser extent, by the corpus luteum of the ovary, and are responsible for the development and maintenance of female secondary sexual characteristics. The other female sex hormone is progesterone, which is also secreted by the corpus luteum; synthetic analogues of progesterone are called progestogens. Progesterone induces the changes required for successful pregnancy.

In non-pregnant females the secretion of oestradiol and the other oestrogens is controlled by follicle stimulating hormone (FSH) from the anterior pituitary gland. Secretion of FSH itself is controlled by gonadotrophin releasing hormone (GnRH) from the hypothalamus. Secretion of progesterone is controlled by luteinising hormone (LH) from the anterior pituitary gland, which in turn is also controlled by GnRH. During pregnancy the oestrogens and progesterone are secreted by the feto-placental unit and their secretion is therefore not controlled by the maternal endocrine system.

Under normal circumstances oestrogens are responsible for the normal physical changes that occur at puberty, for example breast development, fat deposition, female-pattern pubic hair and growth of the long bones of the limbs. Progesterone is responsible for the changes of the endometrium that prepare it for the initiation of pregnancy; progesterone also plays a role in the development of the breasts and lactation. The cyclical secretion of oestrogens and progesterone is also responsible for the endometrial changes that result in regular menstruation.

■ 8.7.1 DISORDERS OF THE FEMALE REPRODUCTIVE SYSTEM AND THEIR TREATMENT

Delayed puberty in females is manifested as primary amenorrhoea, where menstruation never occurs. The cause of primary amenorrhoea may lie in the hypothalamus or anterior pituitary gland or may be at the level of the ovaries. Where the disorder lies at the level of the ovary, the individual can be treated by oestrogen replacement therapy to induce the anatomical changes of puberty, coupled with cyclical progestogens to induce a regular menstrual bleed. In cases of primary amenorrhoea due to hypothalamic or pituitary disorders, menarche may sometimes be induced by administration of a GnRH analogue or an oestrogen receptor antagonist. Oestrogen receptor antagonists such as tamoxifen and clomiphene (clomifene) act by preventing the negative feedback effects of oestrogens and therefore increase the secretion of LH and FSH.

Secondary amenorrhoea is the cessation of normal menstrual cycles. The most common causes are pregnancy and menopause, although factors such as malnutrition and chronic stress may also induce amenorrhoea, as can hyperprolactinaemia (Section 8.8), hyperthyroidism (Section 8.2) and any hypothalamic or pituitary gland disorder. Treatment is by resolution of the underlying disorder, sometimes in combination with clomiphene or tamoxifen therapy.

Another method of inducing ovulation is the administration of analogues of LH and FSH, such as human menopausal gonadotrophin (HMG) or human chorionic gonadotrophin (HCG) or analogues of GnRH. Many women with regular ovulation, however, remain infertile. In some cases of infertility there are anatomical disorders, whereas in others it has been shown that the cervical mucus is 'hostile' to sperm, thus impeding sperm transport, or that the woman is producing anti-sperm antibodies. Another cause of infertility is luteal insufficiency. In this condition the corpus luteum fails to produce sufficient progesterone to maintain the pregnancy until progesterone synthesis is taken over by the feto-placental unit. Treatment is by supplementation with a progestogen during the latter phase of the menstrual cycle until the feto-placental unit develops; non-androgenic progestogens such as dydrogesterone are used to overcome the risks of virilisation of a female fetus. Drug treatments for infertility are summarised in Box 8.3.

Prior to puberty neither oestrogen nor progesterone play any role in development or maturation, thus there are no clinical disorders associated with hormone deficiency. Early exposure to oestrogens, for example due to inappropriate secretion of oestrogens from a tumour, or due to ingestion of exogenous oestrogens can, however, cause premature development of secondary sexual characteristics: precocious puberty. The characteristic

Amenorrhoea may be treated by administration of an oestrogen receptor antagonist

■ *Box 8.3* Some drugs used in the treatment of infertility in males and females

Drug	Proprietary name
Hypothalamic hormones	
Gonadotrophin releasing hormone	HRF®
Pituitary hormones	
Follicle stimulating hormone	Gonal-F®, Puregon®
Human chorionic gonadotrophin (LH)	Pregnyl® (injection), Profasi® (injection)
Human menopausal gonadotrophin (LH + FSH)	Menogon® (injection), Pergonal® (injection)
Oestrogen antagonists	
Clomiphene	Clomid® (tablets),
(clomifene)	Serophaene® (tablets)
Progesterone supplementation	
Dydrogesterone	Duphaston® (tablets)
Dopamine agonist	
Bromocriptine	Parlodel® (tablets)

features of precocious puberty are early development of breasts and pubic hair and an early spurt in linear bone growth. Treatment is by removal of the source of the oestrogens; however, those anatomical changes that occur before treatment are irreversible.

■ 8.7.2 HORMONE REPLACEMENT THERAPY (HRT) AND THE MENOPAUSE

The cessation of menstruation in later life is called the menopause, the most important feature of which is a failure to secrete oestrogens and progesterone. Features of the menopause include periodic feeling of warmth in the head and neck (hot flushes), regression of the female secondary sexual characteristics, for example atrophy of the endometrium and atrophic vaginitis, loss of the protein matrix of the bone (osteoporosis) and cardiovascular disease.

By administration of oestrogens, either transdermally or orally, the hot flushes can be controlled, the regression of secondary sexual characteristics can be inhibited, the onset of osteoporosis can be delayed and the risk of cardiovascular disease reduced by the reduction of plasma cholesterol and low-density lipoprotein (LDL)–cholesterol. However, oestrogen therapy does carry risks, it may promote existing breast cancer and may promote the proliferation of the endometrium or endometrial carcinoma. Oestrogen-only replacement therapy, therefore, is only appropriate for women who have undergone hysterectomy. In women in whom the uterus remains, the risks of endometrial hyperplasia can be decreased by cyclical administration of a progestogen. The administration of a progestogen, followed by its sudden withdrawal, causes a menstrual-like bleed which reduces the risk of the oestrogen-induced endometrial hyperplasia. There is therefore a regular 'period', although this is seen as undesirable by some women. In some cases the progestogen can be given continuously, but irregular bleeding may still ensue.

Some of the orally active progestogens used for the prevention of endometrial hyperplasia possess androgenic properties and therefore produce adverse effects on blood lipids. In these cases the co-administration of the progestogen partially negates the beneficial effects of the oestrogens on the low-density and high-density lipoprotein–cholesterol. The epidemiological data suggest, however, that such combined treatment still offers protection against cardiovascular disease, but not to the same extent as that offered by the use of unopposed oestrogens, but that the cyclical progestogen reduces the risk of endometrial carcinoma to that of an untreated population. There is also evidence that oestrogen replacement therapy may increase the risk of developing breast cancer, although therapy for less than 10 years has no significant effect on the number of breast cancer cases. Progestogens have no effect on the incidence of breast cancer.

Recent advances in hormone replacement therapy have been the introduction of tibolone, which possesses both oestrogenic and progestogenic activity, and drugs with actions on selective subtypes of oestrogen receptors. Tibolone is seen as an advance because it can be used without the need of additional hormone therapy, although its continuous administration means that there are no withdrawal, 'menstrual-like' bleeds, and the selective oestrogen receptor agonists offer the possibility of a beneficial effect on osteoporosis with little or no effect on breast tissue, thus reducing the risk of breast cancer.

■ 8.7.3 ORAL AND OTHER HORMONAL CONTRACEPTIVES

The normal stimulus for ovulation is the mid-cycle surge in LH secretion, thus any treatment that reduces the LH surge is likely to prevent ovulation. Under normal conditions progesterone reduces the secretion of LH by negative feedback, thus administration of exogenous progesterone would be expected to prevent ovulation. Early attempts to test

■ *Box 8.4* Some drugs developed as contraceptives in males and females

	Treatment	Efficacy
Male	GnRH analogue + testosterone	Significantly reduced sperm count in 85% of subjects, no severe adverse effects
	Medroxyprogesterone + testosterone	Significantly reduced sperm count in 90% of subjects, fears of adverse effects of medroxyprogesterone
	Testosterone enanthate	Azoospermia in 58% of users, amongst these 0.8% risk of contraceptive failure per year
Female	Progestogen only	3% risk of contraceptive failure per year
	Combined oestrogen + progestogen	0.3% risk of contraceptive failure per year
	Sequential oestrogen + progestogen	0.3% risk of contraceptive failure per year

this hypothesis used oral administration of natural progesterone; however, because of the high degree of first-pass metabolism of this steroid very large doses were required. The major advance in the development of an acceptable oral contraceptive came with the synthesis of orally active progestogens such as norethisterone (known as norethindrone in USA). Using these synthetic progestogens, which are derived from androgenic steroids, it was shown that it was possible to induce effective, reversible infertility. It is now known that the progestogens act to prevent pregnancy by at least three separate mechanisms: first, the prevention of ovulation, which may not occur in every menstrual cycle; secondly, an increase in the viscosity of cervical mucus, which prevents sperm transport; and, finally, the development of an endometrium into which a fertilised ovum is unable to implant. It is the combination of all of these factors that results in effective contraception.

The progestogen-only oral contraceptive is taken daily, continuously. Typically, the contraceptive efficacy of the treatment is such that there are approximately three pregnancies each year for each 100 users (hundred women years, HWY). This poor contraceptive efficacy is partially due to the fact that the doses of progestogen used do not reliably inhibit ovulation and partially due to the fact that the drug must be taken at the same time each day; it has been suggested that the duration of effect of a single dose of progestogen is barely 24 hours, thus missing the next dose by as little as 3 hours can markedly reduce the contraceptive efficacy. A more recent advance has been the administration of the progestogens by intramuscular injection or subcutaneous implantation. These methods provide 6 weeks to 5 years of contraception from a single administration, and because they overcome the need to take a 'pill' regularly, there are no pregnancies associated with delayed dosing. The most commonly reported problem of progestogen-only contraceptives is irregular, heavy menstruation. The major advantage of these types of contraceptives is their acceptability for use in women who cannot tolerate oestrogens because of an existing underlying disorder, such as a blood clotting disorder. There have also been attempts at targetted delivery of low doses of progestogens directly to the reproductive organs. In one development the progestogen is released from a silicon rubber vaginal ring, in another method the contraceptive effect of an intrauterine device is enhanced by the release of a progestogen from the device.

A later development of oral contraceptives was the addition of an oestrogen to the treatment regime in an attempt to control the irregular, heavy menstruation. This addition of an oestrogen gave rise to the first combined oral contraceptive. Combined oral contraceptives are normally administered daily for 21 days, followed by a 7-day drug-free period. As with the progestogen-only treatment, the combined oral contraceptives reduce fertility by inducing a thickening of cervical mucus and changes in the endometrium, but they are also more effective inhibitors of ovulation. During the 7 drug-free days the withdrawal of the progestogenic support causes endometrial atrophy and therefore a menstrual-like bleed, but contraceptive cover is maintained. The combined oral contraceptives are much more effective than progestogen-only contraceptives, with a theoretical failure rate of approximately 3 pregnancies per 10,000 women per year (0.03 pregnancies per HWY, see later); the regular, predictable 'menstruation' improves user acceptability and provides reliable reassurance that pregnancy has not occurred, but the addition of the oestrogen component increases the risk of adverse effects (see later).

The failure rate of combined oral contraceptives is about 3 pregnancies per 10,000 women per year

In an attempt to reduce the incidence and severity of the adverse effects, lower-dose combined oral contraceptives have been introduced, sometimes by use of regimes where the doses of each of the components are varied throughout the 21 days of treatment, for example the dose of oestrogen may be kept constant whereas the dose of progestogen increases during the middle phase, or the dose of oestrogen may increase for the middle 7 days of treatment whereas the progestogen increases step-wise throughout the whole 21 days (Box 8.4). In addition to the lower total monthly doses, these treatment regimens are believed to mimic the natural menstrual cycle more closely than the single-dose (monophasic) combined oral contraceptives, and are therefore less likely to cause adverse effects.

Oral contraceptives have been associated with a range of adverse effects from chloasma (freckles) to breast cancer. Amongst the less troublesome side-effects are weight gain, breast tenderness and loss of libido, all of which can usually be resolved by changing to a brand of contraceptive with different doses or ratios of oestrogen and progestogen. The most severe of the reported adverse effects, cervical cancer, breast cancer and thrombosis, require greater consideration.

The use of combined oral contraceptives containing high doses (50μg) of oestrogen increases the risk of cervical cancer by 60% after 4–6 years of use and by 100% in women who use them for more than 6 years. It is now recognised, however, that the increased incidence of cervical cancer, a treatable condition, is outweighed by a decrease in the incidence of more serious uterine and ovarian tumours. Similarly, it has been reported that oral contraceptives increase the incidence of breast cancer. It is now believed that the oestrogen component of the oral contraceptives are responsible for an accelerated growth of existing breast tumours, hence use of oral contraceptives increase the likelihood of development of breast cancer before the age of 36; however, overall, oral contraceptives do not increase the total number of breast cancer cases. It is because of this that oral contraceptives should not be used by women with a history of, or an existing, breast tumour.

It is safer to use oral contraceptive for 1 year than to go through one pregnancy

The early, high oestrogen dose, oral contraceptives were associated with an increased incidence of cardiovascular disease, particularly in women over the age of 35 and in women who smoked. This adverse effect has now been reduced following the introduction of lower-dose oral contraceptives and the recommendation that oral contraceptives should be used with care in women over the age of 35 and that oral contraceptive users should not smoke. Currently used oral contraceptives are not associated with increased risk of cardiovascular disease, although some studies have linked certain types of progestogen with an increased risk of deep vein thrombosis, but the risk is still lower than that posed by pregnancy.

■ 8.7.4 OTHER USES OF AGONISTS AND ANTAGONISTS OF OESTROGEN AND PROGESTOGEN RECEPTORS

Other uses for these hormones, and drugs that affect their activity, include fertility control and the treatment of certain hormone-dependent cancers. Oestrogen receptor antagonists can also be used in the treatment of some forms of breast cancer. Approximately 40% of breast tumours are oestrogen-dependent and tumour regression can therefore be induced either by ovariectomy or by use of oestrogen antagonists such as tamoxifen or clomiphene. Oestrogens can also be used in males for the treatment of prostatic carcinoma, an androgen-dependent tumour in males. Progestogens can be used in the treatment of endometriosis, a condition in which endometrial cells proliferate at sites outside of the uterus, and in endometrial cancer.

Oestrogens can also be used for post-coital contraception

High doses of oestrogens can also be used as a post-coital contraceptive. If oestrogens are administered within 72 hours of unprotected coitus, the endometrial environment alters so that implantation cannot occur. A similar approach is to use a progesterone-receptor antagonist such as mifepristone; this agent reduces the supportive effect of progesterone on the endometrium and therefore induces menstruation. An important difference between the post-coital oestrogen contraceptive and the progesterone antagonist is that the former prevents implantation, and therefore prevents pregnancy, whereas the latter causes failure of an established pregnancy.

Side-effects of oestrogens and progesterone range from the severe, such as breast cancer and cardiovascular disease (Section 8.7.3), to the more minor such as nausea and vomiting, fluid retention, headache, breast enlargement and discomfort, weight gain and mood changes for oestrogens, and amenorrhoea, fluid retention, weight gain and increased growth of body hair for progestogens.

■ 8.8 THERAPEUTIC USES OF PITUITARY HORMONES AND THEIR ANALOGUES

The pituitary gland secretes numerous hormones. The posterior portion of the gland secretes antidiuretic hormone and oxytocin, which are discussed in Chapters 5 and 7, respectively, whereas the anterior portion of the gland, which functions independently of the posterior pituitary gland, secretes a further six important hormones. Hormone secretion by the anterior pituitary gland is controlled by the hypothalamus by means of releasing hormones. The majority of the hormones secreted by the anterior pituitary gland are themselves concerned with the control of activity of other glands, thus thyroid stimulating hormone (TSH) controls the activity of the thyroid gland; the gonadotrophins follicle stimulating hormone (FSH) and luteinising hormone (LH) are concerned with secretion of sex hormones in males and females and adrenocorticotrophic hormone (ACTH) controls the secretion of glucocorticoids by the adrenal cortex. The secretion of these pituitary hormones are respectively controlled by thyrotrophin releasing hormones (TRH), gonadotrophin releasing hormone (GnRH) and corticotrophin releasing hormone (CRH) from the hypothalamus. Other hormones from the anterior pituitary gland are growth hormone and prolactin, the secretion of which is again controlled by the hypothalamus. An understanding of the role of the anterior pituitary gland and its relationship with the hypothalamus is important in the understanding of the aetiology of endocrine disorders, the treatment of these disorders and the therapeutic uses of hormones and their analogues, for example a disorder of the reproductive system may be caused by a disease of the gonads themselves, or may be due to a malfunction of the pituitary gland or the hypothalamus. The treatment for such a disorder may therefore be directed at the gonads or at the hypothalamic–pituitary axis, using either analogues of the sex hormones or analogues of FSH, LH or GnRH. The therapeutic uses of GnRH, FSH, LH, ACTH and their analogues have been described in the appropriate sections above. This section will therefore consider only prolactin and growth hormone.

■ 8.8.1 DISORDERS OF PROLACTIN SECRETION AND THEIR TREATMENT

The most common form of anterior pituitary tumour is one which secretes prolactin. Excess secretion of prolactin, hyperprolactinaemia, is associated with a range of symptoms in both men and women. In women the most common symptom is amenorrhoea, whereas in men the presenting symptom is usually infertility. Between a quarter and a half of all female sufferers of hyperprolactinaemia also experience a milky discharge from the breasts. This condition is termed galactorrhoea and it may also occur in up to 30% of male sufferers, although the most common symptoms in males are decreased libido, headache and apathy. Occasionally hyperprolactinaemia may be associated with gynaecomastia (the development of feminine breasts in males). The treatment of galactorrhoea, gynaecomastia and hyperprolactinaemia is usually by administration of the dopamine agonist bromocriptine, although a new drug, cabergoline, has recently been marketed. These drugs act on dopamine receptors in the anterior pituitary gland to inhibit further secretion of prolactin. With both drugs, the most common side-effect is nausea, which is a consequence of the stimulation of dopamine receptors of the chemosensory trigger zone of the medulla oblongata. In some cases the excessive prolactin secretion is a result of drug therapy with drugs that act as dopamine antagonists, the most common group of drugs being the antipsychotic agents (see Chapter 3). The antiemetic drug metoclopramide is also a dopamine antagonist and has thus been seen to cause hyperprolactinaemia.

Hyperprolactinaemia in males, one symptom of which is breast development, can be treated with dopamine agonists

■ 8.8.2 DISORDERS OF GROWTH HORMONE SECRETION AND THEIR TREATMENT

The most important hormone in the control of linear growth is growth hormone (GH) which is secreted under the control of growth hormone-releasing hormone (GH-RH), and to a lesser extent, somatostatin from the hypothalamus. The predominant physiological effect of GH is the promotion of linear growth that occurs during adolescence. This effect results from an increase in protein synthesis and extracellular collagen deposition, which is mediated at the cell nucleus. In children, growth hormone deficiency results in dwarfism. In adults, because normal stature has already been achieved, the growth hormone deficiency has little effect. Treatment of growth hormone deficiency is by hormone replacement therapy but, because of the specificity of the human growth hormone receptor, it is not possible to use growth hormone of animal origin. Early therapies used hormonal material extracted from human cadavers, but recent developments have concentrated on the production of human growth hormone using recombinant DNA techniques, although the resultant products are very expensive. Replacement therapy with these hormones, if initiated before the closure of the epiphyses, may result in extra growth, but many authorities question the cost effectiveness of the treatment as the growth achieved may be as little as an extra 4cm.

Many authorities question the cost effectiveness of growth hormone as it is very expensive and the extra growth achieved may be as little as 4cm

In cases of hypersecretion of growth hormone there is excessive growth; excess before puberty results in gigantism, in which case the symptoms include growth, to a height in excess of 2.5 metres, and increased muscle mass. More commonly the condition presents in adults after normal closure of the epiphyses, when it is characterised by a thickening of the skin around the face, leading to a coarsening of the features and increased growth of the nose and ears. There is also growth of the bones of the skull which results in the development of a jutting jaw and a prominent forehead, the hands and feet also become enlarged, this condition is called acromegaly. Most cases of acromegaly, and gigantism, can be treated with dopamine agonists to stimulate the neuronal pathways that are known to reduce growth hormone secretion, this is succesful in about 70% of cases. More recently is has been possible to administer somatostatin analogues such as octreotide (proprietary name: Sandostatin®) to bring about reduced secretion. In cases where pharmacotherapy is unsuccessful, the tumour is usually removed or destroyed either by surgery or by radiotherapy.

■ SUMMARY

- The endocrine system complements the nervous system in controlling functions such as metabolism, growth and reproduction. The major glands of the system are the hypothalamus, the pituitary gland, the thyroid gland, the parathyroid gland, the pancreas, the adrenal glands and the gonads.
- Treatment of thyroid hormone deficiency is by simple hormone replacement therapy; excessive secretion of the thyroid hormones is treated by surgical removal of the gland or by administration of an inhibitor of thyroid hormone synthesis.
- The parathyroid glands, together with calcitonin and 1,25-dihydroxycholecalciferol (1,25-DHCC) are responsible for calcium homeostasis. Underactivity of the parathyroid gland is treated with 1,25-DHCC; overactivity is treated by promotion of calcium excretion, by use of biphosphonate agents which inhibit bone resorption or by administration of calcitonin.
- The pancreas is responsible for the control of carbohydrate metabolism. A deficiency of the active hormone, insulin, results in diabetes mellitus. If untreated, diabetes mellitus can cause death; treatment is by insulin replacement. Diabetes mellitus may also be caused by loss of response to insulin, this form of diabetes can be treated with oral hypoglycaemic agents.
- The adrenal glands are concerned with the stress response, the inner adrenal medulla secretes adrenaline whereas the adrenal cortex secretes mineralocorticoids and glucocorticoids. An excess of mineralocorticoids results in hypertension, this condition can be treated with an aldosterone antagonist. Excess glucocorticoids cause Cushing's syndrome, the treatment for which is inhibition of the synthesis of the steroid hormones or removal of their source. Underactivity of the adrenal cortex is treated by hormone replacement therapy. Corticosteroids are widely used for the suppression of the immune/inflammatory response.
- The gonads secrete androgens in males and oestrogens and progesterone in females. These hormones are responsible for the initiation and maintenance of secondary sexual characteristics and fertility. Cases of reduced fertility can be treated by replacement of the sex hormones themselves or administration of those pituitary hormones responsible for control of spermatogenesis, ovulation and sex hormone secretion. Lack of ovulation can also be treated with an oestrogen antagonist which reduces the negative feedback

effect. The hormones of the gonads can also be used in males and females to induce reversible infertility, i.e. contraception. The final use for female sex hormones is hormone replacement therapy in post-menopausal women.

- Excessive secretion of the pituitary hormone prolactin causes gynaecomastia in men and infertility in both males and females. Treatment is by administration of the dopamine agonist bromocriptine, which inhibits prolactin secretion.
- Disorders of growth hormone secretion can produce either dwarfism of gigantism. Treatment of growth deficiency is by administration of growth hormone, although only small increases in growth are achieved.

■ REVISION QUESTIONS

For each question select the most appropriate answer. Correct answers are presented in Appendix 1.

1. Carbimazole is used in the treatment of which condition:
   (a) hypothyroidism;
   (b) hyperthyroidism;
   (c) hypoparathyroidism;
   (d) hyperparathyroidism;
   (e) hyperaldosteronism.

2. Oral hypoglycaemic drugs are not used in the treatment of insulin-dependent diabetes mellitus because:
   (a) they produce an excessive decrease in blood glucose concentration;
   (b) they produce an insufficient decrease in blood glucose concentration;
   (c) their side-effects render them unsuitable for use in young patients;
   (d) they require endogenous insulin secretion to produce their effects;
   (e) they only produce their effects in obese patients.

3. Glucocorticoid antagonists are unsuitable for the treatment of Cushing's syndrome because:
   (a) they are unable to cross the target cell membrane;
   (b) they are not orally active;
   (c) they cause rebound excessive secretion of ACTH;
   (d) some authorities see the cost–benefit ratio as being too great;
   (e) none have yet been developed.

4. Which of the following potential side-effects is *not* associated with androgen therapy in females:
   (a) increased muscle mass;
   (b) breast development;
   (c) deepening of voice;
   (d) menstrual irregularity;
   (e) development of male-pattern pubic hair.

5. The failure rate of female combined oral contraceptives is approximately:
   (a) 0.03 pregnancies per 100 women per year;
   (b) 0.10 pregnancies per 100 women per year;
   (c) 0.3 pregnancies per 100 women per year;
   (d) 1.0 pregnancies per 100 women per year;
   (e) 8.0 pregnancies per 100 women per year.

6. Unopposed oestrogen replacement should not be undertaken in post-menopausal women in whom the uterus has not been removed because:
   (a) the uterus is the primary target for the oestrogen therapy;
   (b) the oestrogen therapy may cause endometrial hyperplasia;
   (c) oestrogens are associated with an increased risk of breast cancer;
   (d) progesterone is required for the expression of oestrogen receptors;
   (e) the absence of progesterone potentiates the immunosuppressant effects of the oestrogenic steroids.

■ SELECTED READING

Brody, T.M., Larner, J. and Minneman, K.P. (eds) *Human Pharmacology: Molecular to Clinical* (Third edition), (St. Louis: Mosby), 471–584.

Gard, P.R. (1998) *Modules in Life Science: Human endocrinology*, (London: Taylor & Francis), 33–181.

Rang, H.P., Dale, M.M. and Ritter, J.M. (1999) *Pharmacology* (Fourth edition), (Edinburgh: Churchill Livingstone), 385–463.

THE TREATMENT OF ALLERGIES AND INFLAMMATION

9

■ 9.1 INTRODUCTION

The response of the body to invasion by bacteria, viruses or foreign proteins, or indeed the response to cellular damage, involves an immune or inflammatory response; allergies are immune responses to proteins or other factors not normally considered to be noxious. Inflammation may occur in the absence of an immune response, for example following a nettle sting (see later). The dominant signs of inflammation are pain, swelling, redness, heat and loss of function of the area affected, it can therefore be seen that these signs are features of the symptoms of many illnesses, such as infections, arthritis and asthma. It is not surprising therefore that drugs for the suppression of the inflammatory and immune responses are some of the most commonly prescribed, and the most commonly used over-the-counter medications.

Before considering the mechanisms of actions and clinical uses of the anti-inflammatory agents and the immunosuppressants, it is first necessary to appreciate the processes underlying the immune response and inflammation.

Drugs used for the treatment and relief of inflammation and allergies are some of the most commonly used medicines

■ 9.2 THE PHYSIOLOGY OF INFLAMMATION AND THE IMMUNE RESPONSE

Immunology is a scientific discipline in its own right, and therefore it is not possible to abbreviate all that is known about inflammation and the immune response into one subsection of one chapter of a text of this nature, furthermore immunologists have developed a language of their own which is often incomprehensible to pharmacologists. The following section aims to outline the essential features of the body's chemical defence mechanisms only far enough to enable the understanding of the mechanism of action of the anti-inflammatory and immunosuppressant drugs.

As portrayed in figure 9.1, there are three separate processes by which the body responds to insult. The first series of events are sometimes called innate reactions because they have been identified in most species and are therefore believed to have been developed early in evolution. Cellular damage or challenge results in the synthesis and release of a variety of inflammatory mediators which are generated either within the plasma or within the cells. Examples of such inflammatory mediators are histamine, prostaglandins and leukotrienes; the characteristics of some of the inflammatory mediators are described later. In response to the mediators there is local vasodilation, which increases the blood

• **Figure 9.1** A schematic
representation of the
inflammatory and immune
processes

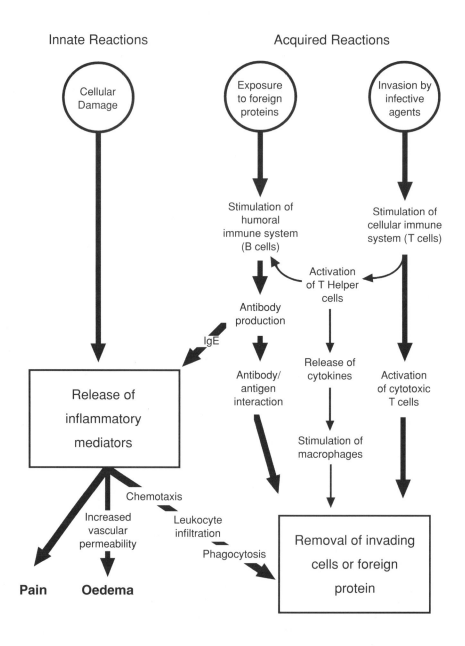

Inflammatory mediators
are responsible for
the cardinal signs of
inflammation: redness,
heat, swelling and pain

flow to the affected area, and increased vascular permeability; these two actions explain the redness, heat and swelling that are features of the inflammatory response. In the case of joints, the swelling also explains the loss of function. The exudate from the capillary not only contains mediators which are able to influence local cells, but, in the case of immune responses, may also contain fragments of the foreign protein or invading organism which are carried to lymphoid tissue where antibody formation is stimulated. Blood cells such as neutrophils and monocytes also migrate out of the blood vessel, attracted by chemotaxins either produced by the invading organism or by adjacent cells, where they engulf the foreign body. Some of the inflammatory mediators also act on local nerve endings to stimulate or facilitate pain sensation.

The other aspect of the body's defence mechanism is the acquired, specific immune process, so called because it requires production of new cells and it is specific for the invading organism or foreign protein; this involves recognition of foreign protein (antigen) by lymphocytes. In the case of the cellular immune system, the T-lymphocytes are either cytotoxic T-cells, so that they attack the invading cells, or else they are T-helper cells which secrete cytokines either to potentiate antibody formation by the B-lymphocytes or to activate macrophages. The B-lymphocytes produce antibodies which interact with the antigen to activate the complement system, which ultimately results in the ingestion or inactivation of the foreign matter. One specific type of antibody, IgE, causes release of inflammatory mediators from mast cells, which therefore explains why most immune events are accompanied by some degree of inflammation.

The immune system plays a vital role in the protection of the individual, but there are times when its actions are inappropriate, examples of such occasions are allergies or hypersensitivities. Allergies and hypersensitivities can be classified into four groups: type I hypersensitivity is when antibodies are produced to non-noxious substances such as grass pollen and foodstuffs. These antibodies are IgE, which cause the release of histamine from mast cells, causing the typical signs such as rhinorrhoea (runny nose) and itch (see below). Type II hypersensitivities are when the antibodies are formed against the host's own tissue, this may follow receipt of donated tissues, for example a blood transfusion, or may be an autoimmune event. Type III and type IV hypersensitivities are when a response is elicited by exposure to a soluble protein to which antibodies have been formed previously, following an initial exposure. The difference between the two are that type III is a more localised response than that of type IV.

■ 9.3 CHARACTERISTICS OF INFLAMMATORY MEDIATORS

Only the major inflammatory mediators will be described but it should be noted that many of these mediators, for example histamine and 5-hydroxytryptamine, also have roles in other aspects of physiology, for example as neurotransmitters and in haemostasis, but only their actions in inflammation will be covered here.

■ 9.3.1 HISTAMINE

Histamine is formed from histidine by the actions of histidine decarboxylase. It is found in most tissues but has particularly high concentrations in the gut, lung and skin. Within the tissues it may be nascent but it is usually found in granules within mast cells, which are similar to the basophils found in the circulating blood. The release of histamine from mast cell granules is precipitated during the inflammatory response, for example by the action of IgE antibodies. Once released, histamine is metabolised by histaminase or by N-methyl-transferase. Interestingly, histamine is also a major component of several insect and plant stings, for example nettle stings.

Histamine is a component of many plant and insect stings

Histamine produces its effects by actions on three receptor subtypes, namely H_1, H_2 and H_3. Histamine H_1, and possibly H_3, receptors utilise inositol triphosphate as their second messenger, whereas the H_2 receptors utilise cyclic adenosine monophospate (cAMP). The function of the receptors is, as yet, not fully understood. H_2 receptors are found in the heart, where they are stimulatory, and in the stomach, where they stimulate gastric acid secretion (see Chapter 7); the important receptors in the inflammatory response are the H_1 receptors. The effect of histamine on the H_1 receptors is to cause contractions of the ileum, bronchioles and uterus; but in blood vessels it causes vasodilation. If histamine is injected intradermally, for example from an insect sting, it elicits what is called the 'triple response'. The triple response consists of a reddening at the site of 'injection', due to local vasodilation, which is surrounded by a wheal. The wheal is the swelling that occurs due to increased vascular permeability, this wheal usually appears paler than the surrounding skin. Surrounding the pale wheal is then the 'flare' which is an area of reddening of the skin; again, this is due to local vasodilation, but in this case it is due to an axonal reflex, rather than a direct effect of histamine. In the nose the increased vascular permeability leads to rhinorrhoea, and widespread histamine release in the skin may cause a rash. Histamine also stimulates nerve endings to cause the sensation of itch. It can therefore be seen that the features of many insect stings can all be attributed to histamine and that, similarly, the symptoms of hay fever are predominantly mediated by histamine.

■ 9.3.2 5-HYDROXYTRYPTAMINE
Like histamine, 5-hydroxytryptamine (5-HT) is found at many sites around the body, predominantly in the gut, the brain and in the platelets. It is synthesised in the gut and brain from the amino acid tryptophan, a dietary amino acid, and is metabolised by monamine oxidase to 5-hydroxyindoleacetic acid; platelets do not synthesise 5-HT but actively take it up within the gut circulation. The actions of 5-HT are mediated by at least seven types of receptor, some of which have two or three subtypes. Overall there are approximately 11 separate sites of action of 5-HT, some of which utilise cyclic adenosine monophosphate (cAMP) as a second messenger, some reduce the formation of cAMP and some act via inositol triphosphate. One subtype, the 5-HT$_3$ receptor, is linked to an ion channel.

The effects of 5-HT are to cause contraction of smooth muscle such as the gut, and to induce vasoconstriction, although some vessels respond to 5-HT by vasodilation, dependent on the receptor subtype present. 5-HT also causes platelet aggregation and stimulates nerve endings to produce the sensation of pain; nettle stings contain a high concentration of 5-HT. 5-HT is also an important excitatory neurotransmitter, see Chapter 3.

■ 9.3.3 EICOSANOIDS
Eicosanoids, of which the prostaglandins are the best known, are not stored but are synthesised 'on demand' from the phospholipid of the cell membrane. The eicosanoids are perhaps the most important mediators of the inflammatory process. The synthetic pathway for the eicosanoids is presented in figure 9.2, with all being derived from arachidonic acid. The initial stage of arachidonic acid liberation is caused by cell damage or following

• **Figure 9.2** The synthesis of the eicosanoids

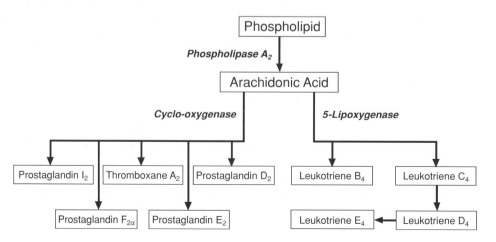

the actions of other inflammatory mediators or of antibodies on mast cells. The actions of the various eicosanoids will be described separately.

9.3.3.1 Prostaglandins

The prostaglandins are formed by the actions of the enzyme cyclo-oxygenase on arachidonic acid. There are two forms of cyclo-oxygenase, labelled COX-1 and COX-2. COX-1 is a normal endogenous enzyme and is present in most cells, COX-2 is said to be inducible, that is, it is only produced under certain circumstances, most notably the inflammatory process. The next stages of the prostaglandin synthesis depend on which cells are involved, for example in platelets the ultimate product is thromboxane-A_2 (TXA_2), in blood vessels it is prostaglandin I_2 (PGI_2 or prostacyclin), in mast cells it is PGD_2 and in macrophages it is PGE_2. Once released, the prostaglandins and thromboxane are rapidly metabolised, with plasma half-lives often being less than 1 minute.

The effects of the various prostaglandins are mediated by specific receptors which have seven transmembrane domains and are coupled to G-proteins, either G_s, G_i or G_q, depending on the receptor. The receptors are named directly from the stimulating agonist, for example PGI_2 acts on IP receptors and TXA_2 acts on TP receptors. Amongst other effects, PGI_2 and PGD_2 cause vasodilation and inhibition of platelet aggregation, TXA_2 causes vasoconstriction and platelet aggregation. These and the other prostaglandins also cause either contraction or relaxation of smooth muscle, inhibition of lipolysis, inhibition of neurotransmitter release and inhibition of gastric acid secretion. During the inflammatory response the prostaglandins are important in producing vasodilation and they potentiate the effects of other mediators, to increase the vascular permeability and increase the stimulation of local sensory pain receptors. They are also involved in the production of the fever that often accompanies infection.

Prostaglandins are produced on demand and are the most important mediators in the production of the components of the inflammatory response, including fever

9.3.3.2 Leukotrienes

Other products of arachidonic acid metabolism are the leukotrienes, which are formed by the actions of the enzyme 5-lipoxygenase which is found in platelets, the lung, mast cells and leukocytes. There are several different leukotrienes (see figure 9.2), and the substance originally named 'slow reacting substance of anaphylaxis' is now known to have been a mixture. Leukotrienes act on specific receptors to induce a range of effects, such as bronchoconstriction, increased vascular permeability and chemotaxis of neutrophils and macrophages. These mediators are released during the inflammatory process and have been found to be particularly prominent in the bronchial and nasal secretions of sufferers of asthma and rhinorrhoea. The new drugs montelukast and zafirlukast are antagonists of the leukotriene C_4 receptor and have been shown to be highly effective for the relief of asthma (see Chapter 6).

Leukotrienes are particularly prominent in the nasal and bronchial secretions of sufferers of rhinitis and asthma

■ 9.3.4 BRADYKININ

Bradykinin is produced by the action of plasma enzymes which become activated following contact with tissues, for example after exudation. Clotting factor XII, Hageman factor (Chapter 5), is one of the factors involved in the production of bradykinin. Following formation, bradykinin is metabolised by kinases, one of which is identical to angiotensin-converting enzyme (Chapter 4), and is found in the lung.

Bradykinin acts on specific receptors, some of which are G-protein coupled, or causes prostaglandin release, to cause vasodilation and increased vascular permeability, contraction of bronchial, intestinal and uterine smooth muscle and stimulation of sensory pain nerve endings.

■ 9.3.5 PLATELET ACTIVATING FACTOR

Platelet activating factor (PAF) is synthesised from phospholipids by phospholipase A_2, the same enzyme that is responsible for prostaglandin and leukotriene production (see figure 9.2). PAF is released from leukocytes following the stimulation that occurs during the inflammatory process. Once released, PAF causes platelets to change shape and to release their contents; this is important in haemostasis (Chapter 5), but it also stimulates synthesis of TXA_2. PAF also causes vasodilation, increased vascular permeability and pain; it can also cause contraction of bronchial and gastrointestinal smooth muscle.

■ 9.3.6 CYTOKINES

The cytokines are a group of mediators which include the interleukins, the interferons, tumour necrosis factors and transforming growth factors. They are synthesised by leukocytes as part of the inflammatory response and they act to enhance the secretion of other mediators, to promote repair processes and to 'overcome' tumour cells and viruses.

■ 9.4 ANTI-INFLAMMATORY DRUGS

There are many conditions in which inflammation is a predominant feature and is the major cause of pain and discomfort. It is because of this that anti-inflammatory drugs are some of the most frequently used. Anti-inflammatory drugs are usually divided into steroidal agents and non-steroidal anti-inflammatory drugs (NSAIDs), although there are other agents, such as antihistamines, which may be of use in reducing inflammation.

■ 9.4.1 STEROIDS

Steroids such as those related to the adrenal glucocorticoid cortisol are potent anti-inflammatory drugs, which also have immunosuppressive properties (see below). In terms of their effects on inflammatory mediators, the most important action is the inhibition of phospholipase A_2, the consequence of which is a reduction in the synthesis of the prostaglandins, thromboxane, the leukotrienes and platelet activating factor. Glucocorticoids also decrease the expression of cyclo-oxygenase (COX-2) and prevent mast cell degranulation; prevention of the generation of cytokines also contributes to the anti-inflammatory effect but also decreases the rate of wound healing and decreases the defence against invading organisms.

> Glucocorticoids are anti-inflammatory because they inhibit phospholipase A_2 and therefore prevent the synthesis of prostaglandins and leukotrienes

Steroidal anti-inflammatory drugs, presented in Box 8.2, are only used when other agents are ineffective or are inappropriate. Steroids are particularly useful in cases of life-threatening inflammatory disorders, when they can be administered intravenously at high doses for 3 consecutive days, the doses can then be reduced and other anti-inflammatory agents introduced. Steroids are also useful for targetted or topical drug delivery, because they are less irritant than other anti-inflammatory agents, thus they can be used for intra-articular injection for the relief of joint inflammation and they are also widely used in the form of creams for the treatment of inflammatory conditions of the skin. Care should be taken when using steroid creams, however; first, because the steroid decreases the defences against infection and therefore increases the risk of infection; and, secondly, because chronic use of steroid creams can cause thinning of the skin. This latter problem also increases the systemic absorption of the topical steroid which could, if excessive amounts of cream were used, lead to adrenal gland suppression (Section 8.5.2.3).

Local administration of steroids to the lungs, in the form of an aerosol inhaler, is a mainstay for the treatment of chronic asthma (see Box 6.4). The steroid is able to prevent the later inflammatory stage of the asthmatic episode, and the local immunosuppression prevents the initiation of the asthma process. The benefit of the local administration is that there is very limited systemic absorption and therefore little risk of adrenal suppression or of any of the other adverse effects of glucocorticoids.

■ 9.4.2 NON-STEROIDAL ANTI-INFLAMMATORY DRUGS

The best known example of a non-steroidal anti-inflammatory drug is aspirin (acetylsalicylic acid), although there are many other common agents, such as paracetamol, which in the USA is called acetaminophen (and actually has no anti-inflammatory properties), and ibuprofen (see Box 9.1). Most of these drugs have three major effects in that they are anti-inflammatory, they are analgesic and they are antipyretic (reduce fever), although the different agents differ in their ability to produce all of the effects. The mechanism of action of these agents is similar in that they all inhibit cyclo-oxygenase and therefore inhibit the synthesis of prostaglandins. Aspirin is an irreversible inhibitor of cyclo-oxygenase, and is relatively selective for COX-1. It has good anti-inflammatory, analgesic and antipyretic properties, but does have adverse effects (see later). Ibuprofen is similarly effective as an analgesic, anti-inflammatory and antipyretic, but is less potent than aspirin and has fewer adverse effects, it has less selectivity for COX-1. Paracetamol has selectivity for COX-1 which is similar to that of ibuprofen, but does not have anti-inflammatory activity, although it is an effective analgesic and antipyretic. One possible explanation for the lack of effect of paracetamol on the inflammatory process is its selectivity for a particular subtype of cyclo-oxygenase which is found in the brain.

Many of the adverse effects of NSAIDs are related to their actions on the gastrointestinal tract. In the stomach, prostaglandins are normally involved in the protection of the gastric mucosa against the corrosive actions of gastric acid; prevention of prostaglandin synthesis by NSAIDs therefore removes this protection and makes the stomach susceptible to irritation and ulceration. This problem is further exacerbated by the fact that many of the NSAIDs are irritant chemicals which, when taken orally, have a direct effect on the gastric mucosa; this problem is partially mitigated by use of dispersed 'soluble' forms

Aspirin prevents prostaglandin synthesis by inhibition of cyclo-oxygenase

---

■ *Box 9.1* Some commonly used non-steroidal anti-inflammatory drugs (NSAIDs)

NSAID	Proprietary name
Aspirin	Various
Indomethacin (indometacin)	Indomax®, Indocid®, Flexin®
Ibuprofen	Nurofen®, Brufen®
Fenoprofen	Fenopron®
Flurbiprofen	Froben®
Ketoprofen	Orudis®, Oruvail®
Fenbufen	Lederfen®
Diclofenac	Diclomax®, Voltarol®
Diflunisal	Dolobid®
Etodolac	Lodine®
Naproxen	Nycopren®, Synflex®
Tenoxicam	Mobiflex®
Tiaprofenic Acid	Surgam®
Sulindac	Clinoril®

of the drug. It has also been suggested that the removal of the protective effects of the gastric prostaglandins is a feature of inhibition of COX-1, and that NSAIDs with selective actions for COX-2 would be effective anti-inflammatory agents, without there being the risk of gastric irritation. Clinical trials to date have failed to support this hypothesis.

Another problem of NSAIDs such as aspirin is their effect on the kidney. Because of the role of prostaglandins in the maintenance of blood flow to the kidney, NSAIDs often cause kidney damage and disorders of salt and fluid balance.

Aspirin has other adverse effects which are not shared by the other members of the group, for example due to effects on haemostasis. As described in Chapter 5, aspirin decreases the risk of thrombosis by inhibiting platelet aggregation; it has been suggested, therefore, that aspirin should not be used for the treatment of dysmenorrhoea (menstrual period pain) because these effects on haemostasis may increase the menstrual blood loss. It is probable that this is only a 'theoretical' effect with very little, if any, increase in the volume of menstrual blood loss, but it is recommended that NSAIDs such as paracetamol or ibuprofen may be the treatment of choice in the relief of dysmenorrhoea. Aspirin can also cause problems in individuals receiving warfarin as an anticoagulant (Chapter 5) as it competes for binding to plasma proteins and therefore increases the effect of the anticoagulant. Aspirin has been associated with Reye's syndrome in children. This is a severe, potentially fatal, disorder of the liver and brain that can follow viral infections. It is because of this association that the use of aspirin is not recommended for children under the age of 12.

The symptoms of aspirin overdose include disturbances of acid–base balance, and a syndrome consisting of tinnitus (a ringing in the ears), dizziness, nausea and vomiting.

The paragraphs above would suggest that aspirin and related substances are highly dangerous substances. This is partially true, and it has been suggested that if aspirin were to be discovered today it would not receive approval for use as a medication, due to the adverse effects, but these effects must be put into perspective: aspirin has been used for hundreds of years and is one of the most effective anti-inflammatory, analgesic, antipyretic agents available. It must also be remembered that use of paracetamol is not free from danger. In overdose paracetamol causes potentially fatal liver damage which develops several days after the paracetamol ingestion. The extent of the liver damage can be limited by increasing the glutathione content of the liver, for example by administration of either acetylcysteine or methionine. As a precautionary measure, paracetamol may be co-formulated with methionine to limit the damage induced by overdose, for example Paradote®.

NSAIDs may also precipitate asthma in susceptible individuals.

Aspirin may not be the best analgesic for the treatment of dysmenorrhoea

■ 9.5 OTHER DRUGS FOR THE RELIEF OF INFLAMMATORY CONDITIONS

The NSAIDs described above limit the pain and oedema of inflammation, but do not treat the underlying condition, nor do they prevent the tissue damage that may accompany long-term inflammation, for example in rheumatoid arthritis. A group of drugs called the disease modifying antirheumatic drugs (DMARDs) have been shown not only to inhibit the inflammatory process, but also to retard tissue damage. Sulphasalazine (sulfasalazine), gold and penicillamine are examples of DMARDs (Box 9.2), a major drawback of these drugs, however, is that they may require up to 6 months' use before any clinical benefit is seen.

The mechanism of action of these agents is unclear but sulphasalasine, gold and chloroquine may act by inhibiting the production of toxic oxygen moieties by leukocytes, thereby inhibiting the cellular damage. Penicillamine reduces the synthesis of the cytokine interleukin-2, as does chloroquine.

■ *Box 9.2* Examples of disease modifying antirheumatic drugs

Class of agent	Drug	Proprietary name
Gold	Sodium aurothiomalate	Myocrisin®
	Auranofin	Ridaura®
Penicillamine	Penicillamine	Distamine®, Pendramine®
Sulphasalazine	Sulphasalazine	Salazopyrin®
(sulfasalazine)	(sulfasalazine)	

■ *Box 9.3* Some common antihistamines used for the treatment of allergy

Class of agent	Drug	Proprietary name	Approximate duration of action
Classical	Azatadine	Optimine®	12 hours
antihistamines	Brompheniramine	Dimotane®	6 hours
	Chlorpheniramine	Piriton®	6 hours
Non-sedating	Acrivastine	Semprex®	8 hours
antihistamines	Cetirizine	Zirtek®	12–24 hours
	Fexofenadine	Telfast®	24 hours
	Loratiadine	Clarityn®	24 hours
	Mizolastine	Mizollen®	24 hours
	Terfenadine	Triludan®	12–24 hours

■ 9.6 ANTIHISTAMINES

The term antihistamine classically refers to antagonists of the histamine H_1-receptor. Because of the prominent effects of histamine released from mast cells as part of the inflammatory process, antihistamines can be used for the relief or prevention of many aspects of the inflammatory/allergic response. Common uses of antihistamines include their systemic use for the prevention or relief of allergies to airborne allergens (e.g. hay fever) or even drug allergies, or as creams for the local relief of the itching induced by skin allergies or insect stings.

Those antihistamines used therapeutically (Box 9.3) differ mainly in their duration of action and profile of adverse effects. The adverse effects of the antihistamines are usually related to effects on receptors other than the H_1-receptor; for example, many antihistamines are also antagonists of the muscarinic acetylcholine receptor, which results in dry mouth, constipation, urinary retention, blurred vision and sedation. Some of these agents are also antagonists at some of the 5-HT receptors, although this usually confers added advantage in the relief of plant and insect stings. The major advance in the treatment of allergies has been the development of long-lasting antihistamines that do not penetrate the blood–brain barrier (see Chapter 10 for discussion of the blood–brain barrier). These allow sustained control of the symptoms of the allergy with reduced risk of sedation, although other antimuscarinic effects may occur.

Sodium cromoglycate (Rynacrom®; Vividrin®) may also be used for the prevention of ophthalmic and nasal allergies and is also used in the prevention of allergic asthma.

Simple antagonists of histamine can relieve the pain and itch of insect stings and prevent the symptoms of allergy

Cromoglycate is not an antihistamine, but prevents the release of histamine from mast cells; it also has effects on cytokines, which may be more important in its role as an anti-asthmatic. Because of its action as a mast-cell stabiliser, cromoglycate does not reverse the symptoms of allergy, but prevents their development. A major drawback of cromoglycate nasal sprays for the prevention of allergic rhinorrhoea is the need to administer the drug 4–6 times daily, in comparison to the nasal steroids, which require twice-daily administration.

■ 9.7 IMMUNOSUPPRESSANTS

Immunosuppressant drugs act to prevent the leukocyte proliferation that occurs during the immune response, and also to prevent antibody formation. Their major uses are to suppress the immune response in autoimmune disorders and also to prevent tissue rejection following organ transplant. Cyclosporin (Sandimmun®) and the related drug tacrolimus (Prograf®) act by preventing cytokine formation and suppressing T-lymphocyte activity, including the stimulatory effects of T-lymphocytes on B-lymphocytes. In addition to their anti-inflammatory properties, glucocorticoids are also immunosuppressant via an effect on cytokine production similar to that of cyclosporin. Both of these groups of drugs have the effect of reducing the white blood cell count and therefore reducing antibody formation.

Immunosuppressants prevent lymphocyte proliferation and antibody production but render the recipient susceptible to infections

Cyclophosphamide (Endoxana®) and azathioprine (Imuran®) are both cytotoxic agents which act selectively in rapidly dividing cells, in this case the rapid proliferation of lymphocytes induced by the immune response. Like the glucocorticoids and cyclosporin (above), these drugs therefore also have the effect of reducing antibody production.

The major clinical problem of all immunosuppressant drugs is that they compromise the body's defences and therefore increase the risk and consequences of infection. The non-cytotoxic immunosuppressants also increased risk of the proliferation of malignant cells.

■ SUMMARY

- Cellular damage or exposure of the body to invading organisms or foreign proteins induces an immune response in which there is leukocyte proliferation and antibody formation; the antibodies act to inactivate the foreign moiety. Parallel to the immune response, and partially independent of it, there is also an inflammatory response which acts to limit the extent of damage following any cellular insult and to initiate the immune response. Inflammation is the predominant symptom of many illnesses and disorders, and therefore anti-inflammatory drugs are some of the most commonly used medicines.
- The inflammatory response is induced by a number of mediators, such as histamine, 5-hydroxytryptamine, prostaglandins and leukotrienes. In general, these act to increase blood flow to the inflamed area, increase vascular permeability and to stimulate the pain sensation.
- The drugs used to relieve or prevent inflammation can be divided into steroids and non-steroidal anti-inflammatory drugs (NSAIDs). Steroids, such as cortisol, act by inhibiting the enzyme phospholipase A_2, which is normally involved in the synthesis of all or many of the inflammatory mediators. NSAIDs act by preventing the actions of the enzyme cyclo-oxygenase, which is involved in the synthesis of the prostaglandin mediators but not in the synthesis of the leukotrienes or platelet activating factor. Drugs of both of these classes are effective in preventing inflammation, but the NSAIDs are also effective analgesics and antipyretics.

- The above-mentioned drugs relieve the symptoms of inflammation but do not treat the underlying cause, nor do they prevent the long-term cellular damage induced by inflammation. Disease modifying antirheumatic drugs (DMARTs) limit the extent of cellular damage induced during inflammation and have been shown to be better than NSAIDs in the treatment of long-term inflammatory conditions such as rheumatoid arthritis, but the effects are slow to onset.

- Antagonists of the histamine H_1-receptor ('antihistamines') are useful in the relief of those symptoms of allergy induced by histamine, for example itch and rhinorrhoea. The adverse effects of these drugs arise from their tendency to antagonise receptors other than the H_1-receptor, most notably the muscarinic acetylcholine receptor. A major advance in the treatment of allergies has been the development of antihistamines with limited ability to cross the blood–brain barrier. Cromoglycate prevents the release of histamine by mast cells and is also of use in the prevention of allergic reactions.

- Immunosuppressant drugs are used to suppress antibody production in autoimmune diseases or following organ transplants. These drugs act to inhibit the synthesis of cytokines or are cytotoxic to the rapidly proliferating lymphocytes. The major adverse effects of these agents is the increased risk and consequence of infection.

■ REVISION QUESTIONS

For each question select the most appropriate answer. Correct answers are presented in Appendix 1.

1. The transduction mechanism for those histamine receptors important in the inflammatory response is:
   (a) stimulation of cyclic AMP synthesis;
   (b) inhibition of cyclic AMP synthesis;
   (c) stimulation of inositol triphosphate synthesis;
   (d) opening of a chloride ion channel;
   (e) opening of a sodium ion channel.

2. The most important action of glucocorticoids in the suppression of the inflammatory response is:
   (a) inhibition of cyclo-oxygenase;
   (b) inhibition of 5-lipoxygenase;
   (c) inhibition of phospholipase C;
   (d) inhibition of phospholipase A_2;
   (e) inhibition of histamine decarboxylase.

3. The most important action of aspirin in the suppression of the inflammatory response is:
   (a) inhibition of cyclo-oxygenase;
   (b) inhibition of 5-lipoxygenase;
   (c) inhibition of phospholipase C;
   (d) inhibition of phospholipase A_2;
   (e) inhibition of histamine decarboxylase.

4. Paracetamol has:
   (a) good anti-inflammatory properties but poor analgesic and antipyretic properties;
   (b) good anti-inflammatory and analgesic properties but poor antipyretic properties;
   (c) good analgesic properties but poor anti-inflammatory and antipyretic properties;

(d) good analgesic and antipyretic properties but poor anti-inflammatory properties;

(e) good antipyretic properties but poor analgesic and anti-inflammatory properties.

5. Terfenadine is less sedating than classical antihistamines because:

(a) it is more selective for the H_1 histamine receptor;

(b) it is a non-competitive antagonist of the H_1 histamine receptor;

(c) it does not penetrate the blood–brain barrier;

(d) it does not penetrate the endothelial barrier;

(e) it is rapidly metabolised by brain decarboxylase.

6. Sodium chromoglycate prevents the symptoms of allergy by:

(a) inhibition of cyclo-oxygenase;

(b) inhibition of phospholipase A_2;

(c) inhibition of histamine decarboxylase;

(d) inhibition of histamine release from mast cells;

(e) antagonism of histamine receptors.

■ SELECTED READING

Galbraith, A., Bullock, S., Manias, E., Hunt, B. and Richards, A. (1999) Nonsteroidal antiinflammatory, antipyretic and analgesic drugs. In Galbraith, A., Bullock, S., Manias, E., Hunt, B. and Richards, A. *Fundamentals of Pharmacology*, (Harlow: Addison Wesley Longman), 336–349.

Kawabata, T.T. (1998) Immunopharmacolgy. In Brody, T.M., Larner, J. and Minneman, K.P. (eds) *Human Pharmacology: Molecular to Clinical* (Third edition), (St. Louis: Mosby), 621–640.

Rang, H.P., Dale, M.M. and Ritter, J.M. (1999) Local hormones, inflammation and allergy. In Rang, H.P., Dale, M.M. and Ritter, J.M. *Pharmacology* (Fourth edition), (Edinburgh: Churchill Livingstone), 198–228.

Rang, H.P., Dale, M.M. and Ritter, J.M. (1999) Anti-inflammatory and immunosuppressant drugs. In Rang, H.P., Dale, M.M. and Ritter, J.M. *Pharmacology* (Fourth edition), (Edinburgh: Churchill Livingstone), 229–247.

■ COMPUTER-AIDED LEARNING PACKAGES

Further details of these learning packages can be found at
http://www.coacs.com/PCCAL/
and
http://cbl.leeds.ac.uk/raven/pha/phCAL.html

Hay Fever and its Treatment (version 2.0), Pharmacy Consortium for Computer Aided Learning (PCCAL), COACS Ltd, University of Bath.

Pharmacology of Inflammation (version 1.96), Pharma-CAL-ogy, British Pharmacological Society, University of Leeds.

APPLIED PHARMACOLOGY

■ 10.1 INTRODUCTION

All of the foregoing chapters have described and discussed the mechanisms of action of medicines, their potential therapeutic uses and their possible side-effects, but this information alone is not sufficient to permit the effective use of those medicines; many other factors must also be taken into account. When drugs are used therapeutically it must be recognised that some drugs have a long duration of action, and therefore repeat dosing needs to be infrequent, and that some drugs have a very short duration of action, which may necessitate very frequent dosing or even continuous infusion. There is also the question of whether the drug can be administered orally, usually the preferred route of administration, or whether it must be injected. Is the drug metabolised by the body? If so, are the metabolites pharmacologically active, inert or toxic? Usually the drug is being used to treat an ill person, does the illness itself alter the activity of the drug, or is that person taking any other medicines? All of these questions, and others, need to be considered. The following chapter aims to illustrate some of the problems associated with the therapeutic use of drugs and some of the factors that should be considered. The first section below will discuss pharmacokinetics and the later sections will discuss some of the other factors.

■ 10.2 BASIC PHARMACOKINETICS

Pharmacodynamics describe the effects of the drug on the body, whereas pharmacokinetics describe the effects of the body on the drug. The four important parameters of the pharmacokinetics of any drug are its absorption, distribution, metabolism and elimination; these four parameters are usually known by the acronym ADME.

ADME: absorption, distribution, metabolism, excretion

■ 10.2.1 FACTORS AFFECTING DRUG ABSORPTION

Most drugs must first enter the body before they can exert any effect. In general terms there are two ways of getting a drug into the body, these are enterally, via the gastro-intestinal tract, or parenterally, for example by injection. In terms of patient satisfaction, the optimum route for drug administration is oral, but several factors may render this impossible. Peptide and protein drugs, for example, may be destroyed by digestive enzymes or by gastric acid, and some drugs are destroyed by gut bacteria. In some cases the drug cannot be given orally because of the effects on the patient; for example, irritant drugs may induce vomiting and diarrhoea or antibacterial agents may have adverse effects on gut bacteria. Examples of drugs that cannot be given orally because of the effects of gastric acid or digestive enzymes are hormones such as insulin and growth hormone or peptide medicines such as vaccines.

Assuming that the drug is able to survive the actions of the digestive system, and is not irritant, the next factor to be considered is whether it will be absorbed. When considering water-soluble drugs it is known that the drugs are more easily absorbed in the gut if they are in their un-ionised form. At the acidic pH of the stomach, weakly acidic drugs are un-ionised and are therefore easily absorbed. Alkaline (basic) drugs will be ionised in acid environments and therefore are not readily absorbed. In the basic environment of the small intestinal, however, the alkaline drugs are un-ionised and therefore absorbed, whereas the acid drugs are ionised and not absorbed. Water-soluble drugs which do not ionise can be absorbed from either site. This process also explains why gastric emptying rate and gastrointestinal motility may influence drug absorbtion. In diarrhoea, for example, gastrointestinal motility is increased, hence the drugs spend less time at the site of absorption and therefore less is absorbed.

Lipid solubility also influences drug absorption. Because the cell membrane is comprised of lipids, lipid-soluble drugs can enter cells more easily than poorly lipid-soluble drugs. One problem with lipid-soluble drugs, however, is that they may become 'trapped' within the lipids of the gastrointestinal contents and excreted without ever being absorbed.

One way to overcome the need to absorb the drug across the gastrointestinal mucosal barrier is to give the drug by injection. Intravenous injections deliver the drug directly into the bloodstream, there is 100% absorption and the drug will become fully diluted within about 2 minutes. One problem of intravenous injection, however, is that immediately after the injection, before the dilution is complete, there will be a local high concentration of the drug within the blood. This local high concentration may be 'toxic' to some tissues, for example heart or brain, and therefore some drugs need to be injected slowly.

Drugs may also be injected intramuscularly or subcutaneously. Muscles have a rich blood supply, thus if the drug is injected into muscle it will diffuse into the capillaries relatively easily and there will be good absorption, over a period of about 30 minutes. Increasing the blood flow to the muscle, for example by exercise, increases the rate of absorption. Drugs may also be injected subcutaneously, this route is less painful than the intramuscular route and is a potential site for self-administration. Because the blood supply to the subcutaneous fat is less than that to muscle, absorption from the subcutaneous site tends to be slower than that from the intramuscular site, although as temperature influences blood flow to the skin it also influences drug absorption. The benefits of these sites of injection are that they remove any risk associated with local high drug concentrations associated with intravenous injection.

One factor that must be taken into account when preparing a drug for injection is the vehicle in which it is injected. Unlike oral administration, where the drug may be administered as a solid, drugs are usually injected in solution, although there are exceptions (see later). For water-soluble drugs this does not present a problem as the drug can be injected either in saline or in water. The closer the injected solution is to being isotonic to extracellular fluid, the less painful is the injection. For lipid-soluble drugs, however, the vehicles are more problematic. Some drugs are injected in dilute ethanol solutions, but this can be painful and, in some cases, the alcohol itself could produce a pharmacological effect. Other vehicles for the injection of lipid-soluble drugs include olive oil and cotton-seed oil. When given intramuscularly, these oily injections produce a depot effect

One way to overcome the need to absorb the drug across the gastrointestinal mucosal barrier is to give the drug by injection

because the drug is more soluble in the oil than in the interstitial fluid. This is used to good effect in the example of injectable contraceptives, where the drug release from a single intramuscular injection may provide contraceptive cover for up to 3 months.

Another form of injection is the solid subdermal implant. These drug-releasing rods are placed below the skin and release their drug over a period of up to 3 months. Such devices are used for the treatment of prostastic carcinoma and for contraception.

Drugs may also be administered by nasal spray. This route is particularly useful if the drug is intended to act only on the nasal epithelium, but can also be used for the delivery of peptide hormones to the bloodstream without them having to go via the gut and the digestive processes. The sublingual route is also a method for avoiding first-pass meta-bolism (see later). Inhalation is also a potential route for the administration of gaseous, volatile or aerosol drugs. In some cases this route is selected because the lungs are the target tissue for the agent, but in other cases, for example general anaesthetics, the mas-sive alveolar surface area of the lungs, with an excellent blood supply, provides a good route for administration of highly lipid-soluble drugs.

The vaginal and uterine routes have also been explored for drug delivery, but obvi-ously in only half of the population. These routes may be used for administration of drugs specifically to these organs, but, in the case of the vagina, the rich blood supply means that drugs placed there may gain access to the systemic circulation.

Local or topical administration of a drug may allow sufficiently high local concentrations to be achieved without the risk of systemic side-effects

The final route of drug administration is the topical route, where the drug is applied directly to the epithelial or mucosal surface on which it is intended to act. Drug absorp-tion from these sites is usually slow, but the locally high concentrations are sufficient to exert a pharmacological effect at the site of application.

With all of these routes of drug administration it must be remembered that the con-dition for which the drug is being administered may itself interfere with the drug ab-sorption. The effects of diarrhoea, vomiting or constipation on oral drug delivery have already been mentioned, but cardiovascular disease may influence blood flow and there-fore influence absorption from the site of injection, and respiratory disease may influ-ence the efficacy of drug administration by inhalation.

■ 10.2.2 FACTORS AFFECTING DRUG DISTRIBUTION

Once inside the body the drug can be distributed either by diffusion or by transport in the blood, but drugs are rarely distributed uniformly. The body should not be consid-ered as a single compartment of fluid throughout which chemicals can distribute, but it should be considered as being multicompartmental. Typically the body fluid may be de-scribed as being comprised of several compartments, the largest of which is the intracellular fluid, this accounts for about 65% of the total body water and is made up of contents of all of the cells of the body. The next largest compartment is the interstitial fluid, which accounts for about 24% of total body water, followed by the blood plasma which accounts for about 8%. Other body fluids, such as the cerebrospinal fluid, intraocular fluid and synovial fluid, make up about 3% of the total body water. The other major fluid compon-ent is fat, which accounts for about 20% of body weight. The distribution of the drug between the various components depends on a number of factors, such as lipid solubility and blood flow to those tissues.

The body is not a single compartment of fluid throughout which chemicals can distribute

Drugs tend to accumulate more rapidly in tissues with a good blood supply, for example the brain, lungs and liver, but with time they may redistribute to the tissues which receive poor blood supply, such as fat. The distribution is also affected by lipid solubility (so that highly lipid-soluble drugs are more likely to accumulate in the brain and, eventually, fat deposits) and by protein binding. Many drugs bind strongly to plasma

• **Figure 10.1** An example
of the calculation of
volume of distribution
for a given drug

Apparent Volume of Distribution

Average plasma volume = 3 litres

Average total body water = 45 litres

$$\text{Apparent volume of distribution} = \frac{\text{Administered dose}}{\text{Plasma concentration}}$$

Give 300mg **mannitol**; plasma concentration = 0.1mg/ml

$$\text{Apparent Volume of Distribution} = \frac{300\text{mg}}{0.1\text{mg/ml}} = 3000\text{ml}$$

This indicates that the mannitol has not left the bloodstream

Give 45g **ethanol**; plasma concentration = 1mg/ml

$$\text{Apparent Volume of Distribution} = \frac{45,000\text{mg}}{1\text{mg/ml}} = 45,000\text{ml}$$

**This indicates that the ethanol has left the bloodstream
and been distributed to all body fluid**

proteins; because the proteins remain largely within the blood vessels, such drugs are seen to remain within the plasma compartment and not to be redistributed. This means that the blood concentrations of the drug remain high, which at first may seem beneficial, but it must be remembered that only the unbound drug is pharmacologically active.

Compartments such as the brain, cerebrospinal fluid and eye are of particular interest. The cells that line the blood vessels supplying these tissues lie in a continuous sheet with tight junctions; the blood vessels supplying other tissues are lined with an incomplete, leaky layer of cells. In order for a drug to penetrate an organ such as the brain, it must either traverse the endothelial cell, which requires high lipid solubility, or it must be transported by a specific transported system, such as the large amino acid uptake system. It can therefore be seen that drug penetration into the brain is selective; this has given rise to the concept of the blood–brain barrier. Interestingly, at times of inflammation the blood–brain barrier may become compromised, this enables the use of systemically administered penicillin, which would not normally cross the blood–brain barrier, for the treatment of bacterial meningitis.

Selective distribution of drugs to the brain gave rise to the concept of the blood–brain barrier

One way to estimate into which compartments a drug has distributed is to consider the volume of distribution. This is a theoretical value, calculated from the plasma concentration of the drug. A sample calculation is presented in figure 10.1. If the volume of distribution is calculated to be 3.5 litres for a given drug, it suggests that the drug is confined to the plasma component. A larger volume of distribution, for example 40 litres, would suggest that the drug is distributed evenly throughout the total body water. If a drug accumulates outside the water compartment, for example by sequestration in fat or by binding to tissues, the volume of distribution exceeds the total body water volume.

■ 10.2.3 DRUG METABOLISM

In the same way that the body normally metabolises foodstuffs to extract the useful substances and to eliminate any toxic components, it also metabolises many drugs. Most of this drug metabolism occurs in the liver, although some occurs in the plasma, lungs or gut. As soon as the drug is absorbed, the concentration of the free drug will begin to decline due to metabolism or excretion (see later). Hepatic drug metabolism is of two kinds, called phase one and phase two. Phase one metabolism involves the disruption of the drug, usually by oxidation, reduction or hydrolysis. This process aims to make the drug chemical more reactive, and in doing so, often makes it more toxic, or even more pharmacologically active. Phase two metabolism is where the 'activated' drug molecule is combined, or conjugated, with another molecule, such as a glucose derivative, to produce a pharmacologically inactive compound, which is usually more water soluble than the original drug chemical.

Most of these chemical transformations are performed by enzymes contained within the cells of the liver. In order for the drug to be metabolised it must therefore first cross the hepatocyte cell membrane. It can therefore be seen that lipid-soluble drugs cross this membrane more easily than, and are therefore metabolised more rapidly than, poorly lipid-soluble (water-soluble) drugs. This gives rise to the statement that 'the process of drug metabolism simply converts lipid-soluble drugs to water-soluble metabolites'.

> The process of drug metabolism simply converts lipid-soluble drugs to water-soluble metabolites

All drugs that are absorbed from the small intestine are first transported to the liver by the hepatic portal vein; in many cases a large proportion of the drug is then metabolised immediately before the drug enters the systemic circulation. The process is called first-pass metabolism. Drugs such as the highly lipid-soluble hormone progesterone undergo extensive first-pass metabolism, such that only about 10% of the administered dose enters the circulation; this is sometimes described as 10% bioavailability. In the case of some drugs, the metabolism occurs within the gut, for example by gut flora, before the drug even reaches the liver; this again is termed first-pass metabolism, with no differentiation being made between hepatic and non-hepatic sites of metabolism. Drugs which are absorbed via other routes, for example by injestion or inhalation, enter the systemic circulation before they reach the liver and therefore avoid first-pass metabolism.

Drug metabolism is usually a first-order reaction, meaning that the rate of metabolism is proportional to the concentration of drug present. This means that as the concentration of drug present is halved, the rate of metabolism is halved; or, expressed in another manner, the time taken to metabolise half of the drug present is constant. This gives rise to the concept of plasma half-life ($T_{1/2}$). For example, if the plasma half-life of a drug is 10 minutes, an initial plasma concentration of $120\mu g/dm^3$ will decrease to $60\mu g/dm^3$ after 10 minutes and to $30\mu g/dm^3$ after another 10 minutes and to $15\mu g/dm^3$ after a total of 30 minutes. Typical plasma half-lives range from a few minutes to days.

> Plasma half-life, the time taken to eliminate half of the amount of drug present, is constant for each drug

In some cases, however, the drug metabolising enzyme may become saturated. In such cases the initial metabolic rate is zero order; that is, a constant rate of so many moles per minute, independent of plasma concentration of the drug, until the drug concentration decreases below the saturation point, when first-order metabolism resumes. An example of this type of biphasic drug metabolism occurs with ethanol.

Hepatic drug metabolism can be complicated by factors such as enzyme induction and enzyme inhibition. Enzyme induction occurs when the liver synthesises more enzyme to cope with the presence of an increased amount of drug. The clinical consequence of this is that, with time, the rate of drug metabolism is increased, and therefore a larger dose of that drug needs to be given more frequently. It is also important to realise that many

> Hepatic drug metabolism can be complicated by factors such as enzyme induction and enzyme inhibition

liver enzymes are able to metabolise more than one drug, thus enzyme induction induced by one drug may lead to increased metabolism of another drug being taken concomitantly. Conversely, if two drugs are metabolised by the same enzyme, addition of a second drug to a treatment schedule may inhibit the metabolism of the first by the process of simple competition.

■ 10.2.4 FACTORS AFFECTING DRUG EXCRETION

Most drug molecules, either unchanged or as metabolites, are excreted via the bile/faeces, urine, sweat or expired air, although some chemicals, for example lead, accumulate within the tissues. As stated earlier, many of the products of hepatic metabolism are water-soluble metabolites of lipid-soluble drugs, these enter the systemic circulation and are transported to the kidney, where they enter the kidney tubule by glomerular filtration. Because the kidney does not possess active transporters for the reabsorption of these metabolites, they are eventually excreted in the urine. In some cases the drug or metabolite avoids glomerular filtration due to binding to plasma proteins. In some of these cases, for example frusemide, the drug is actively secreted into the proximal tubule (Chapter 5). Drugs and metabolites that are in free aqueous solution may also be excreted in sweat or expired air.

Enterohepatic shunt: the process in which the drug is excreted into the gut from the bile duct, but is then reabsorbed and transported back to the liver

Where the drug or metabolite is not freely water soluble, it is normally excreted into the gut via the bile duct, from whence it is excreted in the faeces; this occurs when the drug conjugate has a molecular weight of greater than 450. One complication of this route of excretion is the enterohepatic shunt. In this process the drug is excreted into the gut from the bile duct, but is then reabsorbed and transported back to the liver. The consequence of this is that the presence of the drug or metabolite within the body is extended, which, if the metabolite is pharmacologically active, may extend the duration of action of the drug.

■ 10.2.5 FACTORS AFFECTING PLASMA DRUG CONCENTRATIONS

The actual concentration of drug present within the plasma following administration is dependent on absorption, distribution, metabolism and elimination (excretion). A comparison of the plasma concentrations of a drug following administration of identical doses either by intravenous injection or orally is presented in figure 10.2. Note that only about 50% of the dose administered orally actually enters the circulation and that the plasma half-life of the drug is approximately 3 hours in both cases.

In most therapeutic circumstances drugs are not given as a single dose but as a repeated dose; this has profound effects on the plasma concentrations achieved. Figure 10.3a illustrates the plasma concentrations achieved when the same drug, at the same dose, is given at 3-hourly intervals. Note that the peak plasma concentration achieved is higher than that achieved by the single dose, but that after the initial few doses, the plasma concentrations vary between constant maxima and minima of 20 and $10\mu g/dm^{-3}$ respectively. This state of constant maxima and minima is called 'steady state'.

Increasing the frequency of dosing to once every 90 minutes results in higher plasma concentrations at steady state, with less percentage fluctuation; negligible fluctuation would be achieved with a constant infusion of the drug. Conversely, decreasing the frequency of dosing to once every 6 hours decreases the plasma concentrations at steady state and increases the percentage fluctuations of plasma concentrations. In all cases, steady state is achieved within about four half-lives of the drug (see figures 10.3b and c). In clinical practice, the delay in achieving steady state, therapeutic concentrations is sometimes overcome by giving initial high doses, which are subsequently decreased.

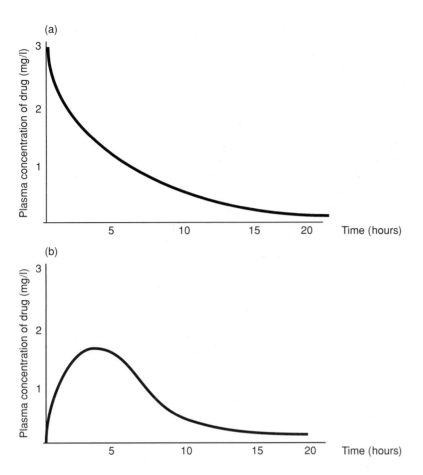

(a)

• **Figure 10.2** Plasma
concentrations of a given
drug after (a) intravenous
or (b) oral administration
of 30mg of the drug

(b)

■ 10.3 INDIVIDUAL VARIATION IN DRUG EFFECTS

The same drug given at the same dose and frequency to two different people may produce quite different degrees of response. The same drug given at the same dose and frequency to the same person on two separate occasions may also produce different responses. The reasons for this may lie in the pharmacokinetics (for example, due to previous food intake causing differences in drug absorption) or they may be pharmacodynamic (for example, changes in receptor populations following repeated use of a drug, see Chapter 1). The diffences may also be due to individual differences between the two recipients, for example age or gender, or due to the disease state. Some of the factors responsible for variation in drug response are described below.

■ 10.3.1 GENDER

There are some obvious examples of gender differences in the responses to drugs, based purely on anatomy (for example oral contraceptives would have a very different effect in males to those seen in females), but there are also gender differences in drug metabolism, especially of steroid hormones. These differences arise because of the presence of different hepatic enzymes that are normally responsible for the metabolism of these hormones.

There are also gender differences in the effects of ethanol. If the same dose of ethanol is given to a male and to a female, the female will normally experience a greater degree of intoxication. This may be due to differences in body weight, but the effect is still present

If the same dose of
ethanol is given to a
male and to a female,
the female will normally
experience a greater
degree of intoxication

• Figure 10.3 Plasma
concentrations of a drug
given at (a) 3-hourly
intervals; (b) 90-minute
intervals; and (c) 6-hourly
intervals

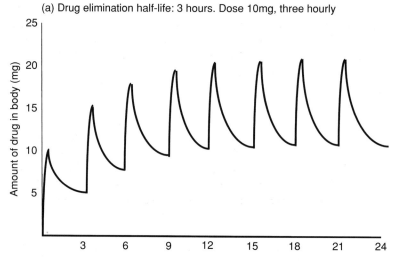

(a) Drug elimination half-life: 3 hours. Dose 10mg, three hourly

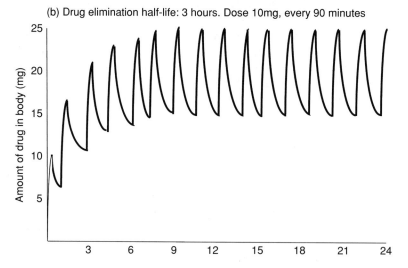

(b) Drug elimination half-life: 3 hours. Dose 10mg, every 90 minutes

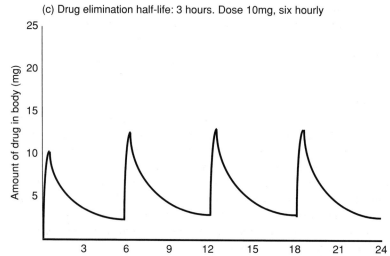

(c) Drug elimination half-life: 3 hours. Dose 10mg, six hourly

if body weight is accounted for by dosing on a 'per kilogram' basis. The reason for this difference is that a greater proportion of a female's body weight is made up of fat. Because fat has a relatively poor blood supply, in females a greater proportion of the ingested dose of alcohol is distributed to the brain than in males, in whom more alcohol is distributed to muscle due to the relatively greater blood supply. This explains the greater degree of intoxication.

■ 10.3.2 AGE
At birth the liver lacks many of the enzymes normally present in the adult, or at least the enzyme activity is very low. In some cases, the adult enzyme activity is achieved within about 8 weeks of birth, but in other cases full enzyme activity is not achieved until adult life. The consequence of this is that some drugs have a much longer plasma half-life in babies than in adults, and that they require a much lower dose, even taking into account the differences in body weight.

At the other end of the scale, liver function also declines with age, which, coupled with the higher body fat content in the elderly, compared with young adults, contributes to the observed extension of the plasma half-life of many drugs in the elderly.

Another factor that contributes to the age-related differences in pharmacokinetics is renal function. Newborn babies have a glomerular filtration rate of approximately one-fifth of that of an adult, although adult filtration rates are achieved very rapidly. As with liver function, renal function also declines with age, with glomerular filtration rate falling by about 50% by the age of 75. This reduction in renal function in the very young and the very old has the effect of decreasing the rate of elimination of many drugs, and therefore increasing the plasma half-life.

■ 10.3.3 INHERITED FACTORS
There are several examples of genetic differences in the ability to metabolise certain drugs. One example is ethanol, which is readily metabolised by Europeans, but poorly metabolised by Chinese subjects, who achieve higher plasma ethanol concentrations. Another example is that of 'acetylator status'. Approximately 50% of the population are described as 'fast acetylators', with the remainder being 'slow acetylators'; acetylation is a common chemical reaction involved in drug metabolism by the liver. There are several other known examples of genetic differences in drug metabolism.

It is also recognised that some populations do not respond to certain forms of therapy. One example of this is the observation that black American hypertensives respond poorly to angiotensin-converting enzyme inhibitors. The reason for this is unclear, but it may be related to ethnic differences in the expression of angiotensin receptors or the converting enzyme.

■ 10.3.4 DISEASE
Any form of liver damage or disease or renal impairment will obviously affect drug elimination, whereas gut disease may influence drug absorption. Pharmacokinetics, however, are not the only reason why disease may alter the response to medication. In some cases of cardiovascular disease, for example, there are changes in the expression of the subtypes of angiotensin receptor, which may influence the efficacy of drugs such as angiotensin-converting enzyme inhibitors or angiotensin receptor antagonists. Similarly, respiratory disorders may cause the development of scar tissue within the lung; scar tissue is unresponsive to bronchodilators. In all cases of disease, the effect of the disease on the action or pharmacokinetics of the drug should be considered.

Whenever two drugs are given together, there is the possibility of a drug interaction

■ 10.4 DRUG INTERACTIONS

Whenever two drugs are given together, there is the possibility of a drug interaction. The term 'drug interaction' refers to the situation where the presence of one drug influences the actions of another. In most cases, the likelihood of a drug interaction can be predicted from a knowledge of the mechanisms of action of the two drugs concerned. Examples of simple receptor-mediated interactions abound. For example, administration of propranolol, a non-selective β-adrenoceptor antagonist, to a hypertensive asthmatic patient who uses salbutamol, a selective β$_2$-adrenoceptor agonist, would not only be expected to precipitate an asthmatic episode but also render the salbutamol inactive. Another example would be the use of L-dopa to treat the extrapyramidal symptoms induced by administration of the antipsychotic agent chlorpromazine, which is a dopamine antagonist. Not only would the L-dopa be likely to lessen the antipsychotic effect of the chlorpromazine, and thereby precipitate a psychotic episode, but the effect of the L-dopa on the extrapyramidal side-effects would be blocked by the presence of the dopamine antagonist.

Additive drug interactions may occur when two drugs with similar effects, not necessarily mediated by the same receptor, are used concurrently; for example, the use of two CNS depressant drugs for two different indications, such as phenobarbitone for the control of epilepsy together with nitrazepam as an hypnotic. The combined effect of the two drugs would be likely to induce severe sedation and loss of co-ordination.

Other forms of drug interaction may involve induction of hepatic enzymes, which increases the rate of metabolism of one of the drugs, or inhibition of enzymes. Similarly, changes in drug distribution and/or elimination may occur if the two drugs compete for the same binding site on a plasma protein, or for a transporter such as that responsible for the transport of amino acids across the blood–brain barrier.

An interesting interaction is that reported between oral contraceptives and antibiotics. Administration of antibiotics results in the reduction of the microbial flora of the gut. Under normal circumstances it is believed that gut bacteria play a role in aiding the absorption of the components of the oral contraceptives, and possibly converting some of the components to more active metabolites. Co-administration of the antibiotic and the oral contraceptive reduces the effects of the gut bacteria and therefore reduces the efficacy of the oral contraceptive.

■ 10.5 THE PLACEBO RESPONSE

No discussion of pharmacology should omit a mention of the placebo effect. A placebo is a treatment which is identical to the active medicine in all characteristics except that it does not contain the active drug. It has been demonstrated many times that if an individual is given a placebo, but told that they are receiving the active drug, there is a high probability that the recipient will report experiencing the effects that would have been expected if they had received the active drug. This has been demonstrated in the relief of many conditions, such as the pain of venepuncture and of tooth extraction and longer-term conditions such as back pain and insomnia; it has also been shown with the effects of alcohol in normal volunteers, where administration of placebo is accompanied by deterioration of psychomotor performance and reports of intoxication. Approximately 30% of the population exhibit placebo responses, and it is often estimated that the size of the effect induced by the placebo is approximately 30% of that expected to have been induced by the active drug. The placebo effect is influenced not only by the information given to the recipient prior to administration, but also by the 'enthusiasm' of the person giving the placebo, the colour of the placebo and the route of administration (oral or injection). The placebo response is greatest in the treatment of conditions with highly subjective symptoms, such as pain and discomfort, mood changes, or changes in the pattern of sleeping, although it has also been observed in conditions such as prostate hypertrophy.

Some authors suggest that the placebo response also contributes to the reported efficacy of several 'active' drugs, the examples cited being the clinical efficacy of antidepressants used at doses well below those recommended, for durations of less than that recommended. Therapeutically, it is believed that the clinician should attempt to enhance the placebo effect whenever a medicine is prescribed.

The converse of the placebo effect is the nocebo effect. This is where the patient reports an adverse effect of a drug following a suggestion made by the prescriber. An example of this would be where a person is warned that a particular medication may cause gastrointestinal disturbances and then subsequently experiences such disturbances, whereas patients who are not warned of the effect do not experience the symptoms.

The importance of an appreciation of the placebo and nocebo effects is that it reminds the pharmacologist that although he or she may be able to predict the effects of a drug precisely under controlled experimental conditions, it is not at all easy to predict the effects of a drug in a human population. It also serves to remind us that although there is much science in modern medicine, there is still a significant degree of 'magic'!

> The placebo response serves to remind us that although there is much science in modern medicine, there is still a significant degree of 'magic'!

■ SUMMARY

- A knowledge of a drug's mechanism of action does not necessarily permit the prediction of the effect of that drug in clinical usage. Some of the most important properties of the drug in relation to its effects are the pharmacokinetic parameters: absorption, distribution, metabolism and excretion.

- Whether a drug is absorbed from the gut is dependent on the degree of ionisation at the different pH values found within the gut (only un-ionised drugs are absorbed effectively) and the lipid solubility. Drugs which are not absorbed orally, or which are degraded by the digestive processes of the gut, may be given by injection, inhalation or by topical application. These local forms of drug administration also have the effect of limiting the extent of the drug effects, and therefore reducing the potential for adverse effects.

- Once absorbed, the drugs are then distributed to the site of action, but distribution is not uniform. Drug distribution to the various components of the body is dependent on the ability of the drug to cross cell membranes, either by utilisation of uptake processes or by simple diffusion, which is dependent on lipid solubility. Other factors that influence drug distribution are the blood flow to the various tissues and the degree of protein binding of the drug.

- From the time the drug first enters the body, the body will attempt to eliminate it. Elimination may be by metabolism or by excretion. Most drug metabolism occurs in the liver in two phases: the first phase renders the drug more reactive, and the second phase then conjugates the drug molecule with another molecule to facilitate excretion via the urine. Many drugs are metabolised before they reach the systemic circulation: first-pass metabolism. The usual route of drug excretion is via the kidneys, although lipid-soluble drugs are excreted via the bile and faeces. Some drugs become 'trapped' by the enterohepatic shunt, where they are excreted via the bile duct back into the gut, only to be reabsorbed and transported again to the liver.

- Other factors that influence the activity of a drug are the gender, age and genetic make-up of the recipients, their state of health and the nature of any other medications they might be receiving. There is also a profound influence of the beliefs and expectations of the individual.

■ REVISION QUESTIONS

For each question select the most appropriate answer. Correct answers are presented in Appendix 1.

1. In the acid environment of the stomach:
   (a) weakly acidic drugs are ionised and therefore not easily absorbed;
   (b) alkaline drugs are ionised and therefore not easily absorbed;
   (c) weakly acidic drugs are un-ionised and therefore easily absorbed;
   (d) alkaline drugs are un-ionised and therefore easily absorbed;
   (e) weakly acidic drugs are un-ionised and therefore not easily absorbed.

2. Which of the following routes of drug administration is least suitable for a peptide drug such as insulin:
   (a) oral;
   (b) intravenous injection;
   (c) intramuscular injection;
   (d) subcutaneous injection;
   (e) nasal spray.

3. An apparent volume of distribution of over 40 litres suggests that:
   (a) the drug remains mainly within circulating plasma;
   (b) the drug is distributed evenly throughout the total body water;
   (c) the drug is extensively protein bound;
   (d) the drug has been redistributed to a non-aqueous compartment;
   (e) the drug does not undergo redistribution.

4. First-pass metabolism:
   (a) is drug metabolism before the drug enters the systemic circulation;
   (b) is drug metabolism as it passes through the systemic circulation for the first time;
   (c) is drug metabolism as it passes through the kidneys for the first time;
   (d) is drug metabolism as it passes through the lungs for the first time;
   (e) is drug metabolism before it passes through the heart for the first time.

5. Phase two drug metabolism:
   (a) makes the drug chemically inert;
   (b) makes the drug more chemically active;
   (c) makes the drug more pharmacologically active;
   (d) makes the drug less pharmacologically active;
   (e) makes the drug more lipid soluble.

6. A drug is said to have reached 'steady state' when:
   (a) it does not undergo further metabolism;
   (b) increasing the dose does not increase the plasma concentration;
   (c) increasing the dosing frequency does not increase the plasma concentration;

(d) the plasma concentrations do not fluctuate;

(e) the plasma concentrations fluctuate between constant limits.

■ SELECTED READING

Galbraith, A., Bullock, S., Manias, E., Hunt, B. and Richards, A. (1999) Pharmacokinetics: absorption and distribution. In Galbraith, A., Bullock, S., Manias, E., Hunt, B. and Richards, A. *Fundamentals of Pharmacology*, (Harlow: Addison Wesley Longman), 73–79.

Galbraith, A., Bullock, S., Manias, E., Hunt, B. and Richards, A. (1999) Pharmacokinetics: metabolism and excretion. In Galbraith, A., Bullock, S., Manias, E., Hunt, B. and Richards, A. *Fundamentals of Pharmacology*, (Harlow: Addison Wesley Longman), 80–91.

Hollenberg, P.F. and Brody, T.M. (1998) Absorption, distribution, metabolism and elimination. In Brody, T.M., Larner, J. and Minneman, K.P. (eds) *Human Pharmacology: Molecular to Clinical* (Third edition), (St. Louis: Mosby), 35–46.

Rang, H.P., Dale, M.M. and Ritter, J.M. (1999) Drug elimination and pharmacokinetics. In Rang, H.P., Dale, M.M. and Ritter, J.M. *Pharmacology* (Fourth edition), (Edinburgh: Churchill Livingstone), 78–92.

Rang, H.P., Dale, M.M. and Ritter, J.M. (1999) Individual variation and drug interaction. In Rang, H.P., Dale, M.M. and Ritter, J.M. *Pharmacology* (Fourth edition), (Edinburgh: Churchill Livingstone), 746–756.

Somogyi, A. (1998) Clinical pharmacokinetics and dosing schedules. In Brody, T.M., Larner, J. and Minneman, K.P. (eds) *Human Pharmacology: Molecular to Clinical* (Third edition), (St. Louis: Mosby), 47–64.

■ COMPUTER-AIDED LEARNING PACKAGES

Further details of these learning packages can be found at
http://www.coacs.com/PCCAL/

Introductory Pharmacokinetics Workshop (version 3.0), Pharmacy Consortium for Computer Aided Learning (PCCAL), COACS Ltd, University of Bath.

Pharmacokinetics Simulations (version 2.0), Pharmacy Consortium for Computer Aided Learning (PCCAL), COACS Ltd, University of Bath.

APPENDIX 1:
ANSWERS TO REVISION QUESTIONS

■ CHAPTER 1

1. The maximal response:
   (d) is that response obtained when an increase in dose produces no increase in response.

2. Antagonists are drugs which:
   (d) bind to the receptor to reduce the actions of the agonist.

3. Some drugs utilise membrane-bound receptors to elicit their response because:
   (d) the drug does not need to cross the target cell wall to produce its effects.

4. Examples of important second messengers involved in hormone actions are:
   (b) IP_3, cAMP, cGMP.

5. G-protein coupled receptors:
   (c) all have similar 'seven transmembrane domain' structures.

6. Which of the following is *not* true about tyrosine kinase receptors:
   (c) tyrosine kinase receptors influence cell differentiation and replication by interacting directly with DNA.

■ CHAPTER 2

1. Which of the following properties is *not* true for the parasympathetic nervous system:
   (c) the neurotransmitter at the neuroeffector junction is noradrenaline.

2. Local anaesthetics act by blocking which of the following:
   (d) voltage-gated sodium ion channels.

3. Which of the following is *not* a form of local anaesthesia:
   (e) central.

4. Which of the following are true of the neuromuscular blocking agent suxamethonium:
   (b) suxamethonium stimulates cholinergic nicotinic receptors at the neuromuscular junction.

5. Which of the following are true of β_1-adrenoceptors:
   (a) β_1-adrenoceptors are found predominantly in the heart.

6. Organophosphate insecticides are:
(d) irreversible inhibitors of cholinesterase.

■ CHAPTER 3

1. Which of the following responses are *not* induced by morphine:
(c) cough.

2. Which of the following explains the anticonvulsant effects of sodium valproate:
(d) blockade of voltage-gated sodium ion channels.

3. Which of the following explains the anxiolytic effects of diazepam:
(c) opening of a ligand-gated chloride ion channel.

4. Which of the following is *not* a potential adverse effect of the antipsychotic agent chlorpromazine:
(d) hypertension.

5. Which of the following groups of drugs would be unlikely to exhibit any antidepressant activity:
(b) decarboxylase inhibitors.

6. A deficiency of which of the following neurotransmitters is believed to be involved in the aetiology of Alzheimer's disease:
(a) acetylcholine.

■ CHAPTER 4

1. Which of the following is *not* a mechanism of action of an antiarrhythmic drug:
(d) chloride ion channel blockade.

2. Cardiac glycosides relieve heart failure by:
(a) inhibition of Na^+,K^+-ATPase.

3. In the relief of angina, glyceryl trinitrate acts by:
(c) increasing nitric oxide concentrations.

4. Angiotensin-converting enzyme inhibitors reduce blood pressure by:
(d) preventing the synthesis of angiotensin II.

5. Which of the following could *not* be used in the treatment of hypertension:
(a) β_2-adrenoceptor antagonists.

6. Which of the following would be expected to elevate blood pressure:
(c) α_1-adrenoceptor agonists.

■ CHAPTER 5

1. Daily, low-dose aspirin therapy is used in prevention of platelet aggregation because:
(b) the irreversible effect of the aspirin lasts for the lifetime of the platelet.

2. Warfarin prevents coagulation by:
(d) preventing the synthesis of factors II, VII, IX and X.

3. Heparin prevents coagulation by:
(b) inhibiting the actions of factors IX, X, XI and XII.

4. Fibrinolytic drugs are used to:
(d) remove the blood clot following coronary thrombosis.

5. Thiazide diuretics act by:
   (d) preventing sodium reabsorption in the distal convoluted tubule

6. The 'statin' lipid-lowering drugs act by:
   (c) preventing synthesis of cholesterol.

■ CHAPTER 6

1. Salbutamol relieves the symptoms of asthma by:
   (c) stimulation of β_2-adrenoceptors.

2. Atrovent® relieves the symptoms of chronic obstructive pulmonary disease by:
   (b) antagonism of muscarinic receptors.

3. Codeine relieves cough by:
   (d) suppressing the cough centre.

4. Ipratropium and oxitropium are used as bronchodilators in preference to other agents that act on the same receptors because:
   (c) they are poorly absorbed and do not cross the blood–brain barrier.

5. The most appropriate treatment for frequent sufferers of asthma is:
   (e) inhaled corticosteroids.

6. Salbutamol is commonly used for the relief of acute asthma because:
   (c) it provides rapid relief.

■ CHAPTER 7

1. The most important mediator in the secretion of gastric acid is:
   (c) histamine.

2. The antiemetic agents most effective against the nausea and vomiting induced by anticancer drugs are:
   (e) antagonists of dopamine (D_2) receptors.

3. In a normal, healthy adult the treatment of choice for acute diarrhoea is:
   (c) fluid replacement.

4. Which of the following would not be used for the treatment of constipation:
   (d) atropine.

5. When used to promote uterine contractions, oxytocin is given by intravenous infusion because:
   (d) it is not absorbed from the gastrointestinal tract.

6. Agonists of which type of adrenoceptors can be used therapeutically to postpone the onset of labour:
   (d) β_2.

■ CHAPTER 8

1. Carbimazole is used in the treatment of which condition:
   (b) hyperthyroidism.

2. Oral hypoglycaemic drugs are not used in the treatment of insulin-dependent diabetes mellitus because:
   (d) they require endogenous insulin secretion to produce their effects.

3. Glucocorticoid antagonists are unsuitable for the treatment of Cushing's syndrome because:
   (e) none have yet been developed.

4. Which of the following potential side-effects is *not* associated with androgen therapy in females:
   (b) breast development.

5. In world-wide use, the failure rate of female oral contraceptives is approximately:
   (c) 0.03 pregnancies per 100 women per year.

6. Unopposed oestrogen replacement should not be undertaken in post-menopausal women in whom the uterus has not been removed because:
   (b) the oestrogen therapy may cause endometrial hyperplasia.

■ CHAPTER 9

1. The transduction mechanism for those histamine receptors important in the inflammatory response is:
   (c) stimulation of inositol triphosphate synthesis.

2. The most important action of glucocorticoids in the suppression of the inflammatory response is:
   (d) inhibition of phospholipase A_2.

3. The most important action of aspirin in the suppression of the inflammatory response is:
   (a) inhibition of cyclo-oxygenase.

4. Paracetamol has:
   (d) good analgesic and antipyretic properties but poor anti-inflammatory properties.

5. Terfenadine is less sedating than classical antihistamines because:
   (c) it does not penetrate the blood–brain barrier.

6. Sodium chromoglycate prevents the symptoms of allergy by:
   (d) inhibition of histamine release from mast cells.

■ CHAPTER 10

1. In the acid environment of the stomach:
   (c) weakly acidic drugs are un-ionised and therefore easily absorbed.

2. Which of the following routes of drug administration is least suitable for a peptide drug such as insulin:
   (a) oral.

3. An apparent volume of distribution of over 40 litres suggests that:
   (d) the drug has been redistributed to a non-aqueous compartment.

4. First-pass metabolism:
   (a) is drug metabolism before the drug enters the systemic circulation.

5. Phase two drug metabolism:
   (d) makes the drug less pharmacologically active.

6. A drug is said to have reached 'steady state' when:
   (e) the plasma concentrations fluctuate between constant limits.

INDEX

metabolism of drugs 151–2
metformin 118
methadone 40, 42
methoxamine 29
methylcellulose 105
α-methyldopa 71
methylprednisolone 105, 121, 122
metoclopramide 104, 105, 107,
    131
metolazone 84
metoprolol 30
midazolam 36, 39
mifepristone 130
milrinone 65
mineralocorticoids 120, 121
mirtazapine 52
moclobemide 51
molgramostim 77
monoamine oxidase 28
    inhibitors 29–30, 50–1, 53
monoamine theory of depression
    50, 54
montelukast 96, 139
morphine 40, 42, 43
    diarrhoea treatment 105, 106
muscarinic receptor antagonists
    32, 53, 94–5, 103, 104, 106
muscarinic receptors 31
myasthenia gravis 27

nabilone 105
nadalol 66
naloxone 43
naproxen 141
nasal sprays 149
nerve blocks 24
nerve impulse, drugs affecting
    23–5
nervous system 21
    see also central nervous system;
    peripheral nervous system
neurodegenerative disorders
    52–4
neuromuscular blockers 25–7, 31
nicorandil 66, 67, 71
nicotine 85
nicotinic acid 87
nicotinic receptors 26, 27
nicoumalone 79
nifedipine 69
nikethamide 92
nitric oxide 61, 71
    donors 66–7
nitrous oxide 36, 38, 39
nizatidine 103
nocebo effect 157
non-competitive antagonism 7–8
non-steroidal anti-inflammatory
    agents 110, 141–2
noradrenaline (norepinephrine)
    27–9, 119
    hypotension treatment 67;
    re-uptake inhibitors 51–2
norethisterone (norethindrone)
    128

occupation theory (drug–receptor
    action) 9
octreotide 132
oestradiol 114, 119, 125
oestrogen replacement therapy
    125–7
oestrogens 124, 125–30
    antagonists 126, 130
omeprazole 103
ondansetron 104, 105
opioid analgesics see narcotic
    analgesics
opioid receptor agonists 36,
    40–41
opioid receptor antagonist 43
opioid receptors 40
oral administration of drugs
    147–8
oral hypoglycaemic agents 118
organophosphates 31–2
orphan receptors 9
osmotic diuretics 5, 82
osmotic laxatives 106
oxytocin 107, 108, 109

pA₂ values 8
pain perception 41–2
pancreatic disorders 116–18
pancuronium 26
paracetamol (acetaminophen)
    141, 142
parasympathetic nervous system
    22, 23, 24
    drugs affecting 31–2
parathyroid hormone 115, 116
Parkinson's disease/parkinsonism
    52–4
penicillamine 142, 143
pentaerythritol tetranitrate
    (pentaerythrityl tetranitrate)
    66, 67
peripheral nervous system, anatomy
    21–3
pethidine 40, 42
phaeochromocytoma 119
pharmocokinetics 147–53, 154
phenelzine 51
phenindione 79
phenobarbitone (phenobarbital)
    43, 44, 45
phenolphthalein 106
phenothiazines 104
phenoxybenzamine 30
phentolamine 30
phenylephrine 29
phenytoin 44, 45
pholcodine 93
phosphodiesterase inhibitors 65,
    71, 95, 118
phospholipase C 15, 16
pilocarpine 31
pirenzepine 103
pituitary hormones and analogues
    130–2
placebo response 156–7

plasma: drug concentration in
    152–3, 154; drugs affecting
    composition 80–7
platelet activating factor 140
platelets 74, 77, 78
polythiazide 84
potassium channels: activator 66,
    67; blockers 63
potassium perchlorate 115
potassium-sparing diuretics 84–5
potency of drugs 4–5
pravastatin 86
prazosin 30, 71
prednisolone 121, 122
prednisone 121
prilocaine 25
primidone 44, 45
Prinzmetal's disease 66
procainamide 62, 63
prochlorperazine 104
progesterone 114, 125, 130
    analogues see progestogens;
    antagonist 130
progestogens 125, 126, 127,
    128–9, 130
prolactin 131
promethazine theoclate 104
propofol 38, 39
propranolol 30, 45, 62, 68–9,
    156
prostaglandins 61, 107, 108–9,
    138, 139
    inhibitors of synthesis 110,
    141–2
prostate cancer 124, 130
proton pump inhibitors 103
pseudoephedrine 29
psychoses 48–50
psychostimulant drugs 30
purgatives 106
pyridoxine (vitamin B₆) 76

quantal responses 3, 4
quinidine 62, 63

ranitidine 103
rate theory (drug–receptor action)
    9
reboxetine 51, 52
receptors 5–6, 8–16
    desensitisation 18, 26;
    intracellular 10–12;
    membrane-bound 10,
    12–16; variations in
    distribution and
    population 17–18; see
    also specific types of
    receptor
red blood cells see erythrocytes
reflux oesophagitis 103
renin–angiotensin system 61, 69,
    70
reserpine 30
respiration 90–1
respiratory depressants 92–3